Current Developments in Stroke

(Volume 2)

(Understanding Stroke in a Global Context)

Edited By

Shanthi Mendis

Geneva Learning Foundation, Former Senior Adviser
World Health Organization, Geneva, Switzerland

General:

1. Any dispute or claim arising out of or in connection with this License Agreement or the Work (including non-contractual disputes or claims) will be governed by and construed in accordance with the laws of the U.A.E. as applied in the Emirate of Dubai. Each party agrees that the courts of the Emirate of Dubai shall have exclusive jurisdiction to settle any dispute or claim arising out of or in connection with this License Agreement or the Work (including non-contractual disputes or claims).
2. Your rights under this License Agreement will automatically terminate without notice and without the need for a court order if at any point you breach any terms of this License Agreement. In no event will any delay or failure by Bentham Science Publishers in enforcing your compliance with this License Agreement constitute a waiver of any of its rights.
3. You acknowledge that you have read this License Agreement, and agree to be bound by its terms and conditions. To the extent that any other terms and conditions presented on any website of Bentham Science Publishers conflict with, or are inconsistent with, the terms and conditions set out in this License Agreement, you acknowledge that the terms and conditions set out in this License Agreement shall prevail.

Bentham Science Publishers Ltd.
Executive Suite Y - 2
PO Box 7917, Saif Zone
Sharjah, U.A.E.
Email: subscriptions@benthamscience.org

**BENTHAM
SCIENCE**

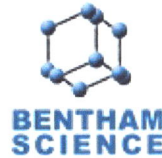

CONTENTS

PREFACE

Stroke is one of the most debilitating major noncommunicable diseases (NCDs). Increasing exposure to behavioural risk factors (tobacco use, unhealthy diet, physical inactivity and harmful use of alcohol) is intensifying the worldwide stroke and NCD burden. The burden of stroke is higher in low- and middle-income countries and, in particular, increasing in the younger age groups. Prevention and management of stroke have advanced a considerably over the last two decades. Scientific advances in the prevention and management of stroke have little value if they are not implemented worldwide. Implementation of new developments for the prevention and management of stroke depends on country resources and capacity that are closely linked to determinants of global health and development.

The world has reached a decisive point in recognizing the interdependence of global health and sustainable development. The agreed Sustainable Development Goals (SDGs), which replaced the Millennium Development Goals (MDGs) in 2015, can only be achieved with the absence of a high prevalence of debilitating diseases such as stroke and other NCDs. At the same time, actions to attain the Sustainable Development Goals can directly or indirectly contribute to reducing the stroke burden. The 17 Sustainable Development Goals relating to future international development include 169 targets to be attained by 2030. They cover a broad range of sustainable development issues, including NCDs. Furthermore, the world has also agreed on a time-bound set of nine voluntary global NCD prevention and control targets to be attained by 2025. The Sustainable Development Goals targets as well as the NCD targets are relevant to stroke. However, there is no clear agreement on *who should do what* to attain these ambitious targets at the country level. What is clear is that multiple actors in many sectors, including health, must work closely together to attain them.

This book is necessary because, at present, there is a serious disconnect between scientific progress in the field of stroke and implementation of these medical advances at the country level. The majority of countries do not adopt a sustainable public health approach to address stroke. A public health approach needs to combine prevention, treatment and monitoring components in order to tackle stroke in a cost effective and sustainable manner. Such an approach also needs to employ an integrated method to address stroke, recognizing that behavioural risk factors of stroke are also responsible for other major NCDs (heart disease, diabetes, chronic respiratory disease and cancer).

Stroke is the field of expertise of neurologists, but combating stroke is the business of everybody. The aim of this book is to introduce and increase the understanding of stroke as well as its links to the Sustainable Development Goals by decision-makers, policy-makers, lay people, journalists, public health practitioners, under-graduate and post-graduate students, and early career-level health professionals working in the fields of stroke, NCDs and development. All of them and others, have a role to play in prevention and control of stroke. A broader understanding of stroke by a wider audience can help to place stroke on the global development and health agenda and to strengthen country capacity to address stroke through a public health approach. There is a need for materials to help equip such interested parties to design, implement and evaluate strategies and programmes to address these diseases. The contents of this book are kept as simple as possible with this need in mind, particularly in the context of low- and middle-income countries.

This book is structured into eight chapters, each addressing key questions on various aspects of stroke. Chapter 1 covers causes, symptoms, signs and consequences of stroke. It has a different style and is much simpler, compared to other chapters, as the aim of this chapter is to introduce stroke to those who have very little knowledge of the condition. Chapter 2 sets out an initial understanding of the sociopolitical and global health landscape, including the competing interests that can render stroke prevention challenging to governments. Chapter 3 discusses stroke and the burden it presents to low-, middle- and high-income countries. It goes on to explore the risk factors and prevention strategies of stroke. Chapter 4 presents the medical and surgical interventions available for managing stroke. Chapter 5 provides an update on the care of stroke, including stroke units, new therapies and future advances. Chapter 6 discusses the links between stroke and the Sustainable Development Goals and is based on information and data obtained from various United Nations documents on Sustainable Development. Chapter 7 presents data on the staggering economic burden of stroke and draws attention to the scarcity of data from the developing world which bears the major share of the global stroke burden. Finally, Chapter 8 summarizes the key messages in simple language. There is some unavoidable overlap between the chapters. The content has been simplified, to the extent possible, to provide better insight and understanding of stroke, particularly to a non-expert audience. It is, therefore, a "must read" for all those interested in stroke and global health.

Prof. Shanthi Mendis
Geneva Learning Foundation,
Former Senior Adviser World Health Organization,
Geneva,
Switzerland

List of Contributors

Bruce C.V. Campbell   Melbourne Brain Centre and Department of Neurology, Royal Melbourne Hospital, Melbourne, Australia

Stephen M. Davis   Melbourne Brain Centre and Department of Neurology, Royal Melbourne Hospital, Melbourne, Australia

Valery L. Feigin   National Institute for Stroke and Applied Neurosciences, Auckland University of Technology, Auckland, New Zealand

Graeme J. Hankey   Department of Neurology, School of Medicine and Pharmacology, The University of Western Australia, Perth, Australia
Department of Neurology, Sir Charles Gairdner Hospital, Perth, Australia
Australia Western Australian Neuroscience Research Institute (WANRI), Perth, Australia

Rita V. Krishnamurthi   National Institute for Stroke and Applied Neurosciences, Auckland University of Technology, Auckland, New Zealand

Peter Langhorne   Academic Section of Geriatric Medicine, Royal Infirmary, University of Glasgow, Glasgow, Scotland

Richard Lindley   University of Sydney, New South Wales, Australia

Shanthi Mendis   Geneva Learning Foundation, Former Senior Adviser World Health Organization, Geneva, Switzerland

Jeyaraj D. Pandian   Department of Neurology, Christian Medical College, Ludhiana, Punjab, India

Priya Parmar   National Institute for Stroke and Applied Neurosciences, Auckland University of Technology, Auckland, New Zealand

Akanksha G. Williams   Department of Neurology, Christian Medical College, Ludhiana, Punjab, India

Current Developments in Stroke

Volume # 2

Understanding Stroke in a Global Context

Editor: Shanthi Mendis

eISSN (Online): 2542-5129

ISSN (Print): 2542-5110

eISBN (Online): 978-1-68108-524-1

ISBN (Print): 978-1-68108-525-8

CHAPTER 1

Stroke: Causes, Symptoms, Signs and Consequences

Shanthi Mendis[*]

Geneva Learning Foundation, Former Senior Adviser World Health Organization, Geneva, Switzerland

Abstract: A stroke occurs when blood flow to the brain is interrupted. The interruption may be due to build-up of fatty deposits on the inner walls of the blood vessels that supply blood to the brain (atherosclerosis and thrombosis), bleeding from a brain blood vessel (haemorrhage) or a blood clot that travels to the brain from a different part of the body (embolus). Cerebral thrombosis, cerebral haemorrhage and cerebral embolism are the three medical terms used to describe these three subtypes of stroke. Common symptoms of stroke include sudden weakness of the face, arm or leg, most often on one side of the body. Tobacco use, harmful use of alcohol, physical inactivity, unhealthy diet and air pollution are the main risk factors of atherosclerosis that lead to stroke. Noncommunicable Diseases (NCDs) (strokes, heart attacks, diabetes, cancer and chronic respiratory disease) share the same risk factors. Long-term exposure to these risk factors also cause raised blood pressure, diabetes and raised blood lipids, which increase the risk of developing strokes. The more risk factors a person has, the greater is the risk of stroke. Nearly two thirds of individuals who develop a stroke die or are disabled. After a first attack of stroke, medicines are required to prevent repeated attacks. Strokes are preventable if individual action is supported by health policies that reduce exposure of people to risk factors. Governments and political leaders have a vital role to play in the prevention of stroke and other NCDs through the implementation of public health policies to control tobacco use, harmful use of alcohol, unhealthy diet, physical inactivity and air pollution.

Keywords: Air pollution, Harmful use of alcohol, Heart attacks, Non-communicable diseases (NCDs), Physical inactivity, Stroke, Tobacco use, Unhealthy diet.

INTRODUCTION

This chapter addresses the following questions.

1. What is a stroke?

---

[*] **Corresponding author Shanthi Mendis:** Geneva Learning Foundation, Geneva, Switzerland; Tel/Fax: 0041227880311; E-mail: prof.shanthi.mendis@gmail.com

2. Can stroke be prevented?
3. How does a stroke develop?
4. What factors increase the risk of a stroke?
5. What other diseases are caused by behavioural risk factors (tobacco use, harmful use of alcohol, unhealthy diet and physical inactivity)?
6. How does a stroke present?
7. What are the consequences of stroke?
8. How is a stroke diagnosed and treated?
9. Can you get repeated attacks of strokes?
10. What is stroke rehabilitation?
11. What can you do to reduce your risk of stroke?
12. What can you do if someone develops features of a stroke?
13. What can governments and political leaders do to improve prevention and care of stroke (NCDs)?

1. WHAT IS A STROKE?

If the blood flow to the brain is interrupted, the brain loses its supply of oxygen and glucose. This causes damage to the brain tissue that is known as a stroke. The World Health Organization (WHO) defines stroke as a clinical syndrome of rapid onset of focal cerebral (brain) deficit, lasting more than 24 hours (unless interrupted by surgery or death) with no apparent cause other than a vascular one [1].

The brain is a vital part of the nervous system that coordinates intellectual, motor and sensory functions of the body. The brain can only function if it is supplied with oxygen and nutrients through its blood supply. Two large blood vessels (known as carotid arteries), which run along either side of the neck, bring blood from the heart to the brain. The blood vessels known as arteries, branch off and become smaller and smaller, until tiny blood vessels supply oxygen, glucose and other nutrients to all parts of the brain (Fig. **1.1**).

Medical terms used to describe stroke include: cerebral haemorrhage; cerebral thrombosis; cerebral embolism; cerebrovascular disease; and transient ischaemic attack. These terms are not interchangeable as they describe different stroke subtypes.

2. CAN STROKE BE PREVENTED?

Stroke is a preventable disease. In 2012, an estimated 6.7 million deaths worldwide were due to stroke. More people die annually from strokes, heart attacks and other preventable diseases of blood vessels (cardiovascular diseases) than from any other cause. Currently, about half (52%) of all premature deaths (deaths under age 70) in the world are due to stroke and other NCDs [2].

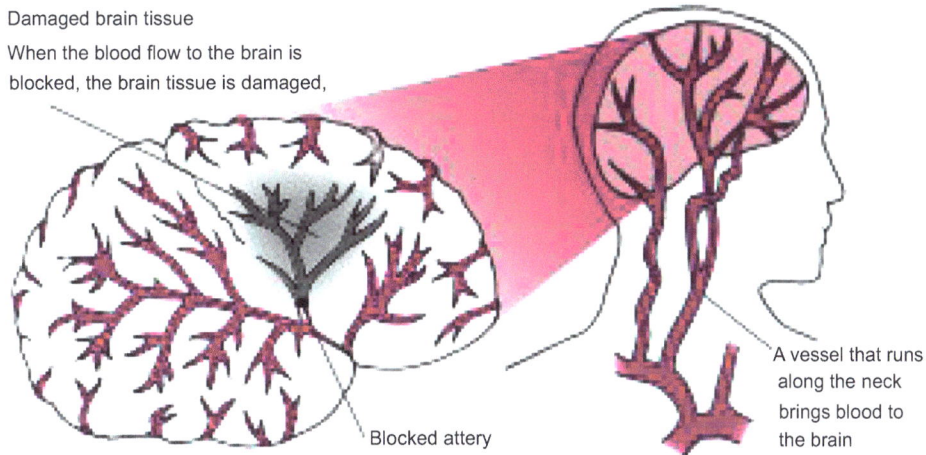

Damaged brain tissue
When the blood flow to the brain is blocked, the brain tissue is damaged,

Blocked attery

A vessel that runs along the neck brings blood to the brain

Fig. (1.1). A stroke happens when the blood supply to the brain is interrupted.
Source: Reprinted from Avoiding Heart Attacks and Strokes. World Health Organization. 2005.

Every year, in addition to 6.7 million people who die from stroke, many more millions are disabled due to strokes. Men as well as women, whether rich or poor, can suffer a stroke. Even when stroke patients have access to modern, advanced treatment, about two thirds die or become disabled. So it is important to know the warning signs and to act fast. But it is even better to prevent strokes from ever happening. Practically all the steps taken to prevent stroke can also prevent heart attacks, as the causative factors of these two diseases are very similar.

3. HOW DOES STROKE DEVELOP?

Strokes are caused by blockage in blood vessels that prevents the flow of blood to the brain. The most common reason for this is a build-up of fatty deposits on the inner walls of the blood vessels that supply the brain. This makes the blood vessels narrower and less flexible (Fig. **1.2**). This process is known as atherosclerosis. When a blood vessel becomes blocked by atherosclerosis the blood supply to an area of the brain is interrupted, and brain tissue is damaged resulting in a type of stroke known as an **ischaemic stroke.** Blood vessels affected by atherosclerosis can also rupture and bleed into the brain causing damage to brain tissue resulting in a type of stroke known as a **haemorrhagic stroke** (Fig. **1.3**). People with raised blood pressure are particularly vulnerable to this type of stroke. Haemorrhagic stroke may sometimes be due to structural abnormalities of blood vessels or brain tumours. Less commonly, blood vessels in the brain can become blocked by blood clots that travel to the brain from elsewhere in the body such as from the heart when it is beating irregularly (this is called atrial fibrillation) This results in a type of stroke known as an **embolic stroke**. In the developed world, 75–80% of strokes are the ischaemic type. The rest are either embolic or haemorrhagic strokes. In the developing world about one third of strokes are of the haemorrhagic subtype.

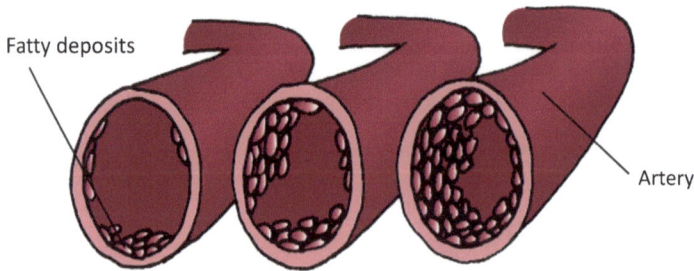

Fatty deposits

Artery

Fig. (1.2). Gradual build-up of fatty deposits along the inside of artery walls (atherosclerosis) leads to narrowing of the arteries.
Source: Reprinted from Avoiding Heart Attacks and Strokes. World Health Organization 2005.

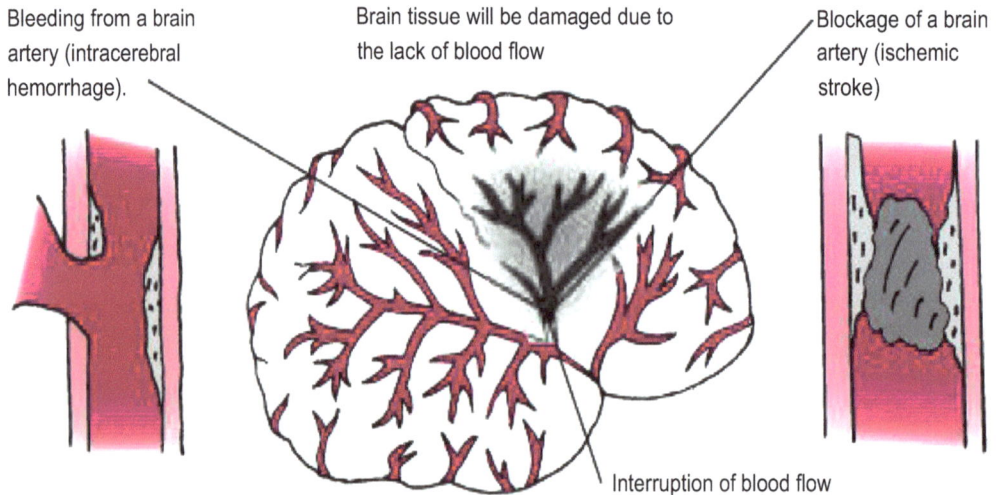

Bleeding from a brain artery (intracerebral hemorrhage).

Brain tissue will be damaged due to the lack of blood flow

Blockage of a brain artery (ischemic stroke)

Interruption of blood flow

Fig. (1.3). Different causes of stroke.
Source: Reprinted from Avoiding Heart Attacks and Strokes. World Health Organization 2005.

There are four main reasons for fatty build-up in blood vessels, all of which can be controlled:

• smoking and other tobacco use;
• following an unhealthy diet too rich in energy, fat and salt; and lack of fruits and vegetables;

- not staying physically active; and
- harmful use of alcohol.

4. WHAT FACTORS INCREASE THE RISK OF A STROKE?

Research shows that a number of things make people more likely to have a stroke (or a heart attack). These are called risk factors. Risk factors may be behavioural, environmental or genetic (Fig. **1.4**). Behavioural risk factors are linked to choices people make. However, improving behaviour is not just an individual problem. Behavioural choices that people make are heavily influenced by knowledge, societal norms and legal and regulatory environments. Genetic susceptibility also plays a role as a risk factor, particularly in people with a family history of stroke in close relatives at a young age.

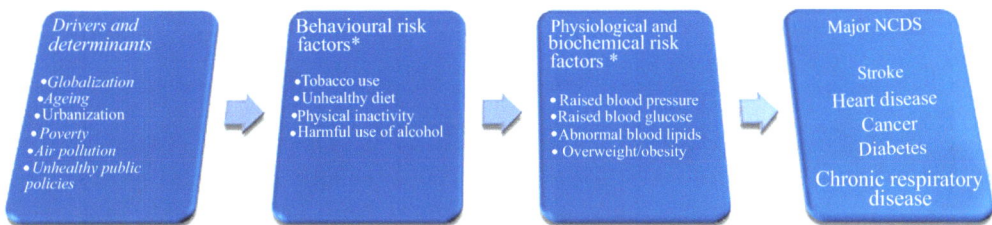

Fig. (1.4). Drivers, determinants and risk factors of stroke and other NCDs.
* Genetic influence can modify the risk.

Governments, policy-makers and politicians have a central role to play in creating conducive environments to help people adopt and maintain healthy behaviours.

The four most important behavioural risk factors are:

- smoking and other tobacco use
- harmful use of alcohol
- unhealthy diet, and
- inadequate of physical activity.

The above unhealthy behaviours cause physical and biochemical changes in the body resulting in other risk factors such as:

- overweight and obesity
- raised blood pressure (hypertension)
- raised blood sugar (diabetes), and
- abnormal blood fats (dyslipidaemia).

These are the most important risk factors for strokes as well as heart attacks. Genetics can play a role in modifying the impact of these risk factors.

Another risk factor of stroke is irregular beating of the heart known as atrial fibrillation. Atrial fibrillation can lead to clot formation in the cavities of the heart. These clots can travel to the brain and block brain blood vessels (cerebral embolism). In developing countries atrial fibrillation is seen even in young age groups in association with rheumatic valve disease of the heart. When atrial fibrillation is not associated with heart valve disease it is mainly seen in the elderly population. With improvements in life expectancy, there is an increased number of elderly people with atrial fibrillation related stroke in both developed and developing countries.

In many parts of the world, tobacco use is on the rise. People are also becoming obese as a result of being less physically active and eating more food that is high in energy (calories), fat and sugar. More young people and children are developing diabetes because they are overweight. There is evidence that prolonged psychological stress can also increase the risk of a stroke or heart attack. People often have more than one risk factor. If a person has two or more of the three risk factors – tobacco use, high blood pressure and high blood sugar – the risk of strokes and heart attacks is greatly increased. The more risk factors, the higher the risk of strokes and heart attacks.

Air pollution is the single most important environmental risk factor. According to WHO estimates, every year 4.3 million deaths occur from exposure to indoor air pollution and 3.7 million deaths occur due to outdoor air pollution [3, 4]. Air pollution is a risk factor for stroke, heart attacks and chronic lung disease and lung cancer. Indoor smoke is a serious health risk for some 3 billion people who cook and heat their homes with biomass fuels and coal. Almost all the deaths due to indoor air pollution are in low- and middle-income countries. Sources of outdoor air pollution include industry, transport, power generation, municipal and agricultural waste management. Most of these sources are well beyond the control of individuals and demand action by policy-makers in multiple sectors, including poverty alleviation, transport, energy and waste management, urban planning and agriculture. While strong cooperation is required between different sectors, health concerns need to be integrated into all national and local air pollution-related policies. Governments have a responsibility to develop systems to monitor air quality and illnesses related to air pollution and promote clean cooking, heating and lighting technologies and fuels and strengthen multisectoral programmes to reduce air pollution.

4.1. Can Tobacco Use Increase the Risk of Stroke?

Tobacco is addictive. Tobacco smoke is full of substances that damage the brain, heart, lungs and blood vessels in the body. These toxic substances take the place of the oxygen in the blood and have the potential to damage all organs causing strokes, heart attacks and cancers. Tobacco also harms babies during pregnancy.

According to WHO, tobacco kills around 6 million people each year. More than 5 million of those deaths are the result of direct tobacco use, while more than 600 000 are the result of non-smokers being exposed to second-hand smoke. Nearly 80% of the world's 1 billion smokers live in low- and middle-income countries. Every person has the right to breathe tobacco smoke-free air. Many developed countries have smoke-free laws to protect the health of non-smokers.

4.2. Can Alcohol Use Increase the Risk of Stroke?

Alcohol is addictive. Harmful use of alcohol can cause stroke, heart attacks, cancer, liver disease as well as injuries resulting from violence and road traffic accidents. Beyond these adverse effects on health of individuals and families, the harmful use of alcohol brings significant social and economic losses to individuals and society at large. According to WHO, 3.3 million deaths every year are resulted from harmful use of alcohol.

4.3. How does the Diet Affect the Risk of Stroke?

An unhealthy diet contributes to strokes, heart attacks, cancers, diabetes and other diseases. An unhealthy diet is one with:

- too much food (too many calories)
- too much fat, sugar or salt, and
- not enough fruit and vegetables

If an individual eats too much food and is not active enough to burn it off, the person will gradually become overweight and obese. Being overweight can lead to diabetes, high blood pressure and high blood fat levels. All of these physical problems increase the risk of heart attacks and strokes. Obese people are at especially high risk if they have a lot of fat around the waist and stomach area. An unhealthy diet often contains too much "fast food", which is high in fat and sugar, and sugar-loaded soft drinks. Fast food is also very high in salt, which increases blood pressure. Recommendations for a healthy diet include eating more fruit, vegetables, legumes (*e.g.* beans and lentils), nuts and grains (*e.g.* brown rice, wheat, millet and oats) and cutting down on salt (*e.g.* less than 5 grams per day or approximately 1 teaspoon per day), sugar and fats. Unsaturated fats (*e.g.* found in fish, avocado, nuts, sunflower, canola and olive oils) are preferable to saturated fats (*e.g.* found in fatty meat, butter, palm and coconut oil, cream, cheese, ghee and lard). Industrial trans fats (*e.g.* found in processed food, fast food, snack food, cookies, margarines and spreads) are not part of a healthy diet.

People are often not aware of the amount of salt they consume. In developing countries people consume too much salt because lot of salt is added to food during cooking, In developed countries, most salt comes from salt added at the table and from processed foods (*e.g.* ready meals, processed meats such as bacon, ham and salami, cheese and salty snacks) or from food consumed frequently in large amounts (*e.g.* bread). Salt is also added to food during cooking, sometimes in the form of stock cubes, soy sauce and fish sauce and also at the table.

Salt consumption can be reduced by:

- reducing the salt added during the preparation of food;
- not having table salt on the table;
- limiting the consumption of salty pickled food and snacks;
- choosing products with lower sodium content; and
- keeping the total daily intake of salt to less than 5 grams (equivalent of 1 teaspoon).

Some food manufacturers are reformulating recipes to reduce the salt content of their products. It is useful to check food labels when purchasing and consuming food products.

4.4. Can Physical Activity Lower the Risk of Stroke?

According to WHO, globally, one in four adults is not active enough. More than 80% of the world's adolescent population is insufficiently physically active. When people do not stay active, their risk of heart attack, stroke, diabetes and cancer increases greatly. Physical activity lowers the risk of these diseases by:

- helping the body burn sugars and fats and keeping an appropriate body weight;
- lowering blood pressure;
- increasing oxygen levels in the body;
- reducing stress;
- strengthening heart muscle, joints and bones; and
- improving blood circulation and muscle tone.

Active people usually have a sense of well-being. They are likely to sleep better and to have more energy, self-confidence and concentration. For example, walking, gardening, cycling or doing housework for at least half an hour a day can help to prevent strokes, heart attacks, cancers and depression.

WHO recommends that:

- children and adolescents aged 5–17 should do at least 60 minutes of moderate to vigorous-intensity physical activity daily; and
- adults should do at least 150 minutes of moderate-intensity physical activity throughout the week.

4.5. Does High Blood Pressure (Hypertension) Increase the Risk of Stroke?

Blood pressure is the force with which the blood pushes against the walls of arteries. The higher the pressure in blood vessels, the harder the heart has to work in order to pump blood. If left uncontrolled, hypertension can lead to heart attack, enlargement of the heart and eventually heart failure. Blood vessels may develop bulges (aneurysms) and weak spots due to high pressure, making them more likely to clog and burst. The pressure in the blood vessels can also cause blood to leak out into the brain. This can cause a stroke. In fact, high blood pressure is the biggest risk factor for strokes. Hypertension can also lead to kidney failure and dementia. Blood pressure is measured in millimetres of mercury (mmHg) and is recorded as two numbers usually written one above the other. The upper number is the systolic blood pressure – the highest pressure in blood vessels and happens when the heart contracts, or beats. The lower number is the diastolic blood pressure – the lowest pressure in blood vessels in between heartbeats when the heart muscle relaxes. Normal adult blood pressure is defined as a systolic blood pressure of 120 mmHg and a diastolic blood pressure of 80 mmHg. All adults need to know their blood pressure and maintain it close to normal levels. Normal levels of both systolic and diastolic blood pressure are particularly important for the efficient functioning of vital organs such as the heart, brain and kidneys and for overall health and well-being.

Hypertension is diagnosed when systolic blood pressure is equal to or above 140 mmHg and/or diastolic blood pressure is equal to or above 90 mmHg. To avoid high blood pressure, people need to stay active, maintain a healthy body weight and eat a healthy diet as described above. If hypertension is diagnosed, then regular medications may be required to keep it under control.

4.6. Does High Blood Sugar (Diabetes) Increase the Risk of Stroke?

Insulin is a hormone produced by a gland in the body known as the pancreas, Insulin helps body cells to use sugar from the blood to produce energy. When the body does not produce enough insulin, or cannot use it properly sugar (glucose) builds up in the blood and results in the development of diabetes. The high blood sugar levels accelerates the development of atherosclerosis – the narrowing and hardening of the arteries. This greatly increases the risk of strokes as well as heart attacks. Raised blood sugar also causes serious damage to many of the body's systems, especially the kidney, nerves and eyes. Treating diabetes involves changing diet and lifestyle. Sometimes, medicines that lower blood sugar are needed.

4.7. Does High Levels of Fat in the Blood (Hyperlipidaemia) Increase the Risk of Stroke?

Blood fats include cholesterol and triglycerides. When there is too much cholesterol and triglycerides in the blood, they cause fatty deposits to build up in arteries, leading to atherosclerosis (the narrowing and hardening of the arteries). This greatly increases the risk of strokes and heart attacks. Cholesterol is not soluble in the blood and is transported attached to particles known as lipoproteins. There are two types of lipoproteins that carry cholesterol to and from cells known as low-density lipoprotein, or LDL, and high-density lipoprotein, or HDL. LDL cholesterol deposits fat in blood vessels and is known as bad cholesterol. HDL cholesterol, helps to remove fat from blood vessels and is known as good cholesterol.

Individuals with cholesterol or triglyceride levels above normal need to eat less fat, stay active and control the body weight. If these measures are not enough, it may be necessary to take medicine to lower the blood fat.

5. WHAT OTHER DISEASES ARE CAUSED BY BEHAVIOURAL RISK FACTORS (TOBACCO USE, HARMFUL USE OF ALCOHOL, UNHEALTHY DIET AND PHYSICAL INACTIVITY)?

Tobacco use, harmful use of alcohol, unhealthy diet and physical inactivity are risk factors for heart attacks, diabetes, cancer and chronic respiratory disease. As these four behavioural risk factors are causative factors of four major diseases, a healthy lifestyle is of paramount importance for protecting good health. Air pollution and poverty also increase the risk of these diseases. Together, they are known as NCDs. Government policies and strategies that assist people to adopt and maintain healthy behaviour and improve the quality of the air people breathe are fundamental for prevention of all NCDs.

6. HOW DOES A STROKE PRESENT?

A stroke usually presents with sudden weakness of the face, arm or leg, most often on one side of the body. Other symptoms include sudden onset of:

- numbness or lack of feeling on one side of the body;
- confusion, difficulty speaking or understanding speech;
- difficulty seeing with one or both eyes;
- difficulty walking, dizziness, loss of balance or coordination;
- severe headache with no known cause; and
- unconsciousness.

The effects of a stroke depend on which part of the brain is affected and how severely the blood flow is interrupted. A stroke may affect just one part of the body such as the face, an arm or a leg or speech. It can also completely paralyse the arm and leg on one side of the body. A very severe stroke can cause sudden death.

About 15% of strokes are preceded by minor strokes known as transient ischaemic attacks (TIA). The features of minor strokes may be similar to those of major strokes, but they are less severe and last only a short time, usually less than an hour. Often, the person recovers without any treatment. These "minor-strokes" are warning episodes; people who have had one or more minor strokes are more vulnerable to develop a major stroke. Minor stroke should not be ignored as medical treatment can prevent the occurrence of a major stroke. A person can have a major stroke without having had any minor strokes.

7. WHAT ARE THE CONSEQUENCES OF A STROKE?

The consequences of a stroke depend on the part of the brain affected and the extent of damage. Severe strokes are associated with serious loss of function, long-term problems and disabilities. They include:

- problems with movement of limbs due to muscle weakness or paralysis, usually on one side of the body;
- problems with feeling (sensation) on one side of the body;
- problems with balance, coordination and walking;
- impaired memory, ability to speak, read and write;
- impaired control of bladder and bowels; and
- psychological and cognitive problems
- coma and death.

The amount of long-term disability depends on how much lasting brain embolic the stroke caused. Many stroke survivors are left with mental and physical disabilities. Those who become paralysed as a result of a stroke need special supportive care in hospital to help them recover and to avoid long-term disability. Most patients who have a stroke are left with some physical disability and may need rehabilitation and long-term care at home including physical and psychological support from family and friends to help them cope.

8. HOW IS A STROKE DIAGNOSED AND TREATED?

The level of medical care for stroke can vary from place to place, depending on the availability of resources and the organization of the health system. The amount of care required depends on the severity of the stroke. In many settings, if the patient reaches a hospital within four and a half hours after the first sign of a stroke, then a thrombolytic medicine can be given to dissolve any blood clots in the brain. However, thrombolytic therapy is for carefully selected patients with acute ischemic stroke. The choice of treatment will depend on the exact type and cause of the stroke. Haemorrhagic strokes are caused by bleeding into the brain due to rupture of a blood vessel. In many cases, this is associated with high blood pressure. To diagnose the type of stroke, certain information is needed, including history, examination findings and results of various tests such as electro-cardiography, computerized tomography (CT) and magnetic resonance imaging (MRI). These tests will help to diagnose whether a stroke is an ischaemic stroke (caused by a blockage of a blood vessel) or a haemorrhagic stroke (caused by a burst blood vessel in the brain). In hospitals with advanced facilities special surgical procedures can be done to minimize the damage to the brain (see Chapter 4). In addition, as discussed in Chapters 4 and 5 dedicated stroke units have been shown to improve the outcome of strokes. Thrombolytic therapy, special surgical procedures for treatment of acute stroke and stroke units are not available in many less-developed countries. Even when these interventions are available the cost is unaffordable for the majority of people in low- and middle-income countries. Prevention of stroke is, therefore, extremely important, particularly in countries with weak health systems.

9. CAN YOU GET REPEATED ATTACKS OF STROKE?

Yes. Almost one third of strokes occur in those who have previously had a stroke. A person who has had a stroke is extremely susceptible to developing another stroke. Before discharge from hospital advice needs to be given on adopting healthy behaviours, including quitting tobacco, reducing harmful use of alcohol, engaging in regular physical activity and following a healthy diet.

Certain medicines are prescribed to prevent first-time strokes and recurrent strokes. Medicines used to treat and manage strokes include:

- antiplatelet agents, such as aspirin;
- anticoagulants or blood thinners, such as warfarin;
- medicines to control blood pressure, such as calcium-channel blockers,

angiotensin converting enzyme inhibitors, beta-blockers and diuretics;
- medicines to lower blood fats, such as statins; and
- medicines to control irregular heartbeat (atrial fibrillation).

These medicines must be used under medical supervision. Aspirin, blood pressure and blood sugar lowering agents and statins to prevent first and recurrent strokes can be made available in primary care even in resource constrained settings. Anticoagulants (such as warfarin), although effective in preventing embolic stroke in people with atrial fibrillation, require regular blood tests to monitor the level of anticoagulation. Most primary care facilities in developing countries do not have facilities for such monitoring. Although there are newer anticoagulants that do not require close monitoring, currently, they are unaffordable to most patients in developing countries.

10. WHAT IS STROKE REHABILITATION?

Stroke rehabilitation is a process undertaken with the active participation of the patient and others to reduce the impact of the disease and disability on daily life. Rehabilitation attempts to restore patients as close as possible to their pre-illness physical, mental and social capability. Stroke rehabilitation includes:

- teaching patients how to exercise safely and effectively;
- helping to manage daily chores, such as walking, eating, dressing, bathing, cooking, reading, writing and going to the toilet;
- speech therapy to help regain normal speech;
- occupational therapy to help patients stay active;
- physiotherapy to help regain movement;
- checking to ensure that patients can live safely at home;
- providing assistance for psychology and mood
- helping to organize medical and rehabilitative care;
- counselling patients and families to enable them to cope better with the stroke.

11. WHAT CAN YOU DO TO REDUCE YOUR RISK OF STROKE?

There is so much that individuals can do to reduce the risk of stroke. Actions taken to reduce the risk of stroke will also prevent heart attacks:

- quit the use of tobacco and avoid inhaling smoke from other people's cigarettes;
- quit or limit the use of alcohol;
- spend at least half an hour a day doing something active, such as walking, cycling, gardening or housework;
- eat five servings (400 grams) of fruit and vegetables each day and limit salt (less than 1 teaspoon or 5 grams per day), fat and sugar in the diet;

- have a periodic health check to check weight, blood pressure, blood fats and blood sugar, particularly after age 40; and
- know your numbers and keep them at desirable levels – *e.g.* blood pressure 120/80 mmHg; fasting blood glucose between 4–6 mmol/L; blood cholesterol less than 5.2 mmol/L; HDL cholesterol/cholesterol between 3.5–1; body mass index: weight (kilograms)/height (metres^2) 18.5-24.9 kilograms/metres^2.
- If you have already had a stroke, take medical treatment to prevent a repeat attack of stroke.

12. WHAT CAN YOU DO IF SOMEONE DEVELOPS FEATURES OF A STROKE?

As described above, sudden inability to speak or sudden weakness of the face, arm or leg on one side of the body or sudden difficulty in walking and coordination are signs of a stroke. If you see someone showing these signs of a stroke, call for medical assistance or an ambulance immediately, or take the person to the emergency department of the nearest hospital. This should be done even if the symptoms are not very severe, because a minor stroke is a warning signal that a person is at increased risk of stroke.

13. WHAT CAN GOVERNMENTS AND POLITICAL LEADERS DO TO IMPROVE PREVENTION AND CARE OF STROKE (NCDS)?

Governments and political leaders play a critical role in prevention and control of stroke (NCDs). Perceptions regarding the health and economic costs of stroke (NCDs), public demand and responsibility for the problem all influence their responses. Policy decisions that have a bearing on stroke (NCDs), made by elected and appointed officials in various ministries such as finance, trade -and agriculture are influenced more by political factors than concerns for health of the people. As discussed in Chapter 2, weak governance, fiscal constraints and resistance from commercial interests often lead governments to adopt incremental policy changes that are too weak to create conducive environments that can transform the behaviour of people.

Very little has been done at the international level, to inform high level decision makers of the devastating individual consequences and the colossal microeconomic and macroeconomic impact of stroke. Information on stroke disseminated through high quality scientific journals dealing with stroke, such as "Cerebrovascular Diseases" or "Stroke", have remained limited to professionals. It is true that certain types of acute stroke if diagnosed within hours, can be treated with thrombolysis or mechanical clot retrieval. However, in reality, these treatment modalities are too sophisticated and expensive to be widely delivered through the fragile and under-resourced health systems of most developing countries. In low income countries, if at all, acute stroke interventions may be available only in one or two tertiary care hospitals in the capital cities. Even then, weak public transport systems particularly in the peripheral regions of these countries, prevent majority of acute stroke victims from accessing treatment in a timely fashion. For these reasons, stroke care with a credible global perspective has to prioritize prevention and rehabilitation, domains which are much less in need of sophisticated means, and costly teams and units.

There is room to accelerate efforts to address stroke worldwide [5, 6]. All countries need to integrate prevention and control stroke (NCDs) within the national response to attain sustainable development goals (see Chapter 6). Gaps in prevention and care of stroke are most notable in low-and middle-income countries. In low-income countries with resource constraints, available resources have to be invested in very cost effective interventions to make stroke prevention and care more efficient and equitable (see Table **1.1**).

Table 1.1. Minimum requirements for prevention and control of stroke in low and medium resource settings

Components	Low Resource Settings *e.g.* Low Income Countries	Medium Resource Settings
Determinants of health (see Chapter 6)	Integrate prevention and control of stroke (NCDs) in the national response to attain SDGs, prioritizing SDG goals 1 and 3	Integrate prevention and control of stroke (NCDs) in the national response to attain SDGs
Risk factors (see Chapters 2, 3 and 4)	Implement policies to attain global NCD targets on tobacco, harmful use of alcohol, population salt consumption and physical inactivity	Implement policies to: - attain global NCD targets on tobacco, harmful use of alcohol, population salt consumption and physical inactivity - reduce exposure to an unhealthy diet - attain NCD targets on diabetes and hypertension -reduce air pollution
Prevention in high risk people (see Chapters 2,3 and 4)	Improve access to early detection and treatment of high risk people to prevent first and recurrent strokes and to attain global NCD target 8, at least in the population above 40 years of age	-Improve access to early detection and treatment of high risk people to prevent first and recurrent strokes and to attain global NCD target 8 -Improve early detection and stroke prevention in people with atrial fibrillation
Health system Governance (see Chapters 2, 3 and 4)	-Increase resources for prevention of stroke (NCDs) -Strengthen primary health care to implement primary and secondary prevention of stroke	-Increase resources for prevention of stroke (NCDs) -Strengthen primary health care, acute stoke care, stroke unit care and stroke rehabilitation

(Table 1.1) contd.....

Components	Low Resource Settings *e.g.* Low Income Countries	Medium Resource Settings
Health financing (see Chapters 2,3 and 4)	-Invest more resources to address stroke (NCD) prevention and control -Include primary and secondary stroke prevention interventions in basic benefit package (*e.g.* WHO Package of Essential NCD interventions, WHO PEN)	-Invest more resources to address stroke (NCD) prevention and control -Facilitate phased-out provision of financial protection for stroke prevention and care - Improve access to affordable sustainable stroke unit care -Advance towards Universal Health Coverage
Service delivery (see Chapters 2,3, 4 and 5)	-Provide basic acute stroke care: Recognition of stroke symptoms and admission to health facility for basic blood tests *e.g.* blood glucose, assessment of swallowing and management to prevent infection, aspiration pneumonia, dehydration hypoglycaemia, deep vein thrombosis and skin ulcers -Implement primary and secondary prevention of stroke through primary health care approach (global NCD target 8 and WHO Package of Essential NCD interventions, WHO PEN)	-Provide emergency unit care diagnosis, investigations including neuroimaging and thrombolytic therapy for acute stroke -Deliver acute stroke care in stroke units -Implement primary and secondary prevention of stroke through primary health care approach (global NCD target 8) -Provide access to stroke rehabilitation services with early functional assessment, goal setting, individualized rehabilitation and follow-up plans
Technologies and medicines (see Chapter 2)	Improve access to basic technologies and medicines listed in global NCD target 9	Improve access to diagnostic lab tests, electrocardiography, echocardiography and neuroimaging and medicines including those listed in global NCD target 9
Health workforce (see Chapters 4 and 5)	-Provide education and skills training to those involved in stroke care including those at first contact level -Train in risk factor assessment, total cardiovascular risk approach, management, basics of acute stroke care and rehabilitation and secondary prevention	-Provide education and skills training to those involved in stroke care including those at first contact level -Train in risk factor assessment, total cardiovascular risk approach, management, basics of acute stroke care and rehabilitation and secondary prevention -Improve access to physicians with expertise in acute stroke care, stroke prevention and rehabilitation -Train interdisciplinary teams for stroke unit care and rehabilitation

(Table 1.1) contd.....

Components	Low Resource Settings *e.g.* Low Income Countries	Medium Resource Settings
Health information systems (see Chapters 2, 3, 4 and 5)	-Improve accuracy of systems for registering births and deaths -Establish population risk factor surveillance -Gather reliable health information for NCDs (stroke) using integrated approaches in primary health care	-Improve accuracy of systems for registering births and deaths -Establish population risk factor surveillance -Gather reliable health information for NCDs (stroke) using integrated approaches in primary health care -Establish hospital based stroke registries -Establish audit systems to improve quality of stroke care and outcomes
Families and communities (see Chapters 4 and 5)	Train patients and families in early recognition of stroke, simple rehabilitation techniques and self-management	Improve access to: -home care stroke rehabilitation services - organized outpatient stroke rehabilitation services -organized family and community support groups
Research and development (see Chapter 7)	Conduct context specific research to investigate: - how to implement what has worked in other settings, in resource constrained contexts -how to implement very cost effective stroke prevention and control interventions *e.g.* WHO best buy NCD interventions -the microeconomic and macroeconomic impact of stroke	Conduct context specific research to investigate: -how to implement cost effective stroke prevention and control interventions -the microeconomic and macroeconomic impact of stroke -

CONCLUDING REMARKS

Stroke is a devastating disease which is prevalent worldwide. Even when stroke patients have access to modern, advanced treatment, about two thirds of them die or become disabled. So it is important for people to know the symptoms and signs of stroke and to act fast. The best course of action is to prevent strokes from ever happening. Evidence based action to combat stroke can be taken even in resource constrained settings. Practically, all the steps taken to prevent stroke also prevent heart attacks and other major NCDs because the causative factors and determinants of these diseases are similar. Governments have the responsibility to integrate efforts to address stroke (NCDs) within the national response to attain SDGs and to adopt a public health approach to prevent and control stroke.

CONFLICT OF INTEREST

The author declares no conflict of interest, financial or otherwise.

ACKNOWLEDGEMENTS

Ms AvisAnne Julien is thanked for copy-editing.

REFERENCES

[1]   Hatano S. Experience from a multicentre stroke register: a preliminary report. Bull World Health Organ 1976; 54(5): 541-53.
[PMID: 1088404]

[2]   World Health Organization. Global health estimates: deaths, disability-adjusted life year (DALYs), years of life lost (YLL) and years lost due to disability (YLD) by cause, age and sex, 2000–2012. Available at: http://www.who.int/healthinfo/global_burden_disease/estimates/en/

[3]   World Health Organization. Burden of disease from the joint effects of household and ambient air pollution for 2012. 2014. Available at: http://www.who.int/phe/health_topics/outdoorair/databases/AP_jointeffect_BoD_results_March2014.pdf

[4]   World Health Organization. Global Health Observatory data: household air pollution. Available at: http://www.who.int/gho/phe/indoor_air_pollution/en/

[5]   World Stroke Organization. Roadmap for delivering quality stroke care 2016. Available at: http://www.world-stroke.org/education/2016-12-19-10-55-24/roadmap-to-delivering-quality-stroke-care

[6]   Mendis S, Davis S, Norrving B. Organizational update: the world health organization global status report on noncommunicable diseases 2014; one more landmark step in the combat against stroke and vascular disease. Stroke 2015; 46(5): e121-2.
[http://dx.doi.org/10.1161/STROKEAHA.115.008097] [PMID: 25873596]

CHAPTER 2

Stroke, Politics, Global Health and Development

Shanthi Mendis[*]

Geneva Learning Foundation, Former Senior Adviser World Health Organization, Geneva, Switzerland

Abstract: At present, there is a serious disconnect between medical advances in the field of stroke and its worldwide application. Implementation of new advances to treat stroke depends on country resources and capacity. Stroke (NCDs) cannot be prevented if exposure to risk factors is ignored and action is taken only to provide high technology treatment for strokes. Prevention of first and recurrent attacks of stroke in high risk people through a primary health care approach and affordable stroke unit care for stroke victims need to be prioritized. Governments have a responsibility and a fundamental role to play in prevention by protecting people from exposure to tobacco, harmful use of alcohol, unhealthy food and air pollution. Effective implementation of policies to reduce exposure to behavioural risk factors and air pollution is challenging and is often influenced by politics. The tobacco, alcohol and food industries use devious tactics to protect profits at the expense of the health of people. The general public could lobby to support government policies that protect the health of people.

Keywords: Air pollution, Behavioural risk factors, Governments, Harmful use of alcohol, Non-communicable diseases (NCDs), Obesity, Physical inactivity, Public health policies, Stroke, Tobacco use, Unhealthy diet.

INTRODUCTION

This chapter addresses the following questions:

1. Why has the global burden of stroke (NCDs) got out of hand?
2. How powerful are the forces driving the stroke (NCDs) burden?
3. What are the tactics used by industry to undermine government policies to prevent stroke?
4. Do children and other vulnerable groups need protection from stroke (NCDs)?
5. Are governments doing enough to prevent childhood obesity?
6. What are the challenges that slow down the prevention and control of stroke (NCDs)?

[*] **Corresponding author Shanthi Mendis:** Geneva Learning Foundation, Geneva, Switzerland; Tel/Fax: 0041227880311; E-mail: prof.shanthi.mendis@gmail.com

7. Is government action matching the size and complexity of the stroke (NCDs) burden?
8. What kind of country action is essential for the prevention of stroke (NCDs)?
9. What could governments do to reduce the exposure of people to behavioural risk factors of stroke (NCDs)?
10. How can health systems be strengthened for cost-effective prevention and control of stroke (NCDs)?
11. Does the global health and development milieu support action of governments?
12. Should governments be held accountable for inaction?

1. WHY HAS THE GLOBAL BURDEN OF STROKE (NCDS) GOT OUT OF HAND?

Major NCDs (stroke, heart attacks, diabetes, chronic respiratory disease and cancer) are diseases that are driven by profits, power, politics and demographic and epidemiological change. As discussed in Chapter 3, since 1990, there has been a steady increase in the absolute number of strokes, and the number of deaths from stroke. The global stroke (NCDs) burden has got out of hand due to inadequate attention to three modifiable causes. First, powerful forces that drive the stroke burden have been allowed to undermine public health policy using various tactics. Second, governments have failed to overcome these forces and implement multisectoral policies to reduce the exposure of people to behavioural risk factors (tobacco, alcohol, unhealthy diet and physical inactivity). Third, primary health care has not been strengthened for effective early detection and treatment of people at risk of developing stroke.

Exposure to behavioural risk factors can be reduced if governments take action to shape and regulate the social, economic and physical environments that people live in. Unhealthy behaviour causing stroke (NCDs) entails the use of strongly addictive substances such as tobacco and alcohol. A characteristic feature of addictive behaviour is the pursuit of immediate satisfaction at the risk of longer-term adverse outcomes. Consequently, people become addictive before they have an opportunity to exercise consumer choice. Although individual action is important for the prevention of stroke (NCDs), a supportive environment is critical for adopting and maintaining healthy behaviour.

2. HOW POWERFUL ARE THE FORCES DRIVING THE STROKE (NCDS) BURDEN?

The forces driving the stroke (NCDs) burden are very powerful. Globalization of marketing and trade has led to the dominance of large multinational corporations that make money from tobacco, alcohol and unhealthy food. Global governance is weak and regulations are practically non-existent to match the growing power and influence of multinational corporations, which wield enormous economic and political influence and have massive marketing promotion budgets. For example, in 2008, the five major United States of America cigarette companies spent US$ 9.94 billion on marketing cigarettes in the country alone [1], an amount surpassing the gross domestic product (GDP) of at least 50 developing countries. Some of these countries still do not even have a dedicated unit within the Ministry of Health to address NCDs [2]. Most of the others have just one health professional to deal with the myriad challenges and complexities of handling the control of tobacco, alcohol and unhealthy diet. This unequal power and resource distribution has profound implications on national responses to combat NCDs in developing countries and makes it difficult for them to withstand industry tactics that undermine national law making. Not surprisingly, most low- and middle-income countries are lagging behind in developing and implementing policies to control unhealthy consumption behaviours [2].

Currently, the marketing strategies of the tobacco industry are primarily targeting vulnerable populations, including children and women. Their main focus is on less-developed countries with weaker regulatory frameworks [3]. More recently, the tobacco industry has even challenged the sovereign authority of states to protect health through tobacco control in Australia, Canada, India, Namibia, Nepal, Norway, the Philippines, South Africa, Sri Lanka, Togo, Turkey, the United Kingdom of Great Britain and Northern Ireland, Uruguay and the European Union [4 - 6]. In some of these countries, the tobacco industry is contesting pictorial health warnings and plain packaging as a tobacco control strategy, arguing that the packaging regulations impinge upon trademark and intellectual property rights. Some of these cases are pending. The majority of these governments, however, have won the legal battle to uphold national tobacco control measures. Behind most of these examples, there are courageous politicians who have put their political careers at risk to provide leadership to take on big tobacco. Former Health Minister Nicola Roxon of Australia, former President of Uruguay Tabaré Ramón Vázquez Rosas and Health Minister Rajitha Senaratne of Sri Lanka are three examples. There are many others (Table **2.1**). Courageous actions of such politicians should give other politicians greater confidence, conviction and courage to fight the tobacco menace.

The alcohol industry is also powerful. The value of alcohol marketing worldwide is estimated at US$ 1 trillion [7]. There is growing evidence that the alcohol industry is also using tactics somewhat similar to the tobacco industry to avoid any form of regulatory and legislative control [8 - 12].

Table 2.1. Presidents, Prime Ministers and Ministers of Health who have received World Health Organization awards for their accomplishments in tobacco control.

Year	Awardees
2004	Micheál Martin TD, Minister for Health and Children, Ireland *
2005	Khandaker Mosharraf Hossain - Minister Health and Family Welfare, Bangladesh
2006	Kyaw Myint, Minister of Health, Myanmar
2007	Ginés González García, Minister of Health, Argentina*
2008	Ary Ibrahim, Ministerof Health, Niger
2009	Rudolf Zajac, Minister of Health of the Slovak Republic, Slovakia
2010	Tabaré Vázquez, President of the Oriental Republic of Uruguay, Uruguay*
2011	Ary Ibrahim, Minister of Health, Niger
2012	Elena Salgado Méndez, Minister of Health, Spain
2013	Ramadoss, Minister for Health and Family Welfare, Government of India*
2014	Maksim Cikuli, former Minister of Health, Albania
2015	Nimal Siripala de Silva, Minister, Health, Democratic Socialist Republic of Sri Lanka
2016	Denzil Douglas, Prime Minister of St Kitts and Nevis*
	Arthur Owen, Former Prime Minister of Barbados*
	Patrick Manning, Prime Minister of Trinidad and Tobago*
	Umar Aliyu Moddibo, Former Minister, Federal Capital Territory, Nigeria
	Mondher Zenaidi, Minister of Public Health, Tunisia
	Recep Tayyip Erdoğan, President of Republic of Turkey*
	Moushira Khattab, Minister of Family and Population Affairs, Egypt
	George A. Papandreou, Prime Minister of Greece*
	Nicola Roxon, Minister for Health and Ageing, Australia
	Lyonpo Zangley Dukpa, Minister for Health, the Kingdom of Bhutan
	Aminath Jameel, Minister of Health and Family, the Republic of Maldives
	Jurin Laksanawisit, Minister of Public Health, the Kingdom of Thailand
	Andrei Usatîi, Minister of Health, the Republic of Moldova
	Karim Massimov, Prime Minister of the Republic of Kazakhstan
	Chen Zhu, Minister of Health, People's Republic of China
	Marziye Vahid Dastjerdi, Minister of Health the Islamic Republic of Iran
	Endang Rahayu Sedyaningsih, Minister of Health, the Republic of Indonesia
	Pradit Sintavanarong, Minister of Public Health, the Kingdom of Thailand*
	Recep Tayyip Erdoğan, President of the Republic of Turkey
	Viktor Orbán, Prime Minister of Hungary
	Maithripala Sirisena, Minister of Health, the Democratic Socialist Republic of Sri Lanka
	Nafsiah Mboi, Minister of Health, Republic of Indonesia
	Gurbanguly Berdimuhamedov, President of Turkmenistan
	James Reilly, Minister of Health, Republic of Ireland
	Iurie Leanca, Prime Minister of Moldova
	Saira Afzal Tarar, Minister of State for Health Services, the Islamic Republic of Pakistan
	Richard Nchabi Kamwi, Former Minister of Health, the Republic of Namibia
	Chris Baryomunsi, Minister of State for Health, the Republic of Uganda
	Daniel Ortega Saavedra, President of Nicaragua
	Tabaré Vázquez, President of Uruguay
	Ilir Beqaj, Minister of Health, Albania
	Surendra Singh Negi, Cabinet Minister of Health, State of Uttarakhand, Republic of India

(Table 2.1) contd.....

Year	Awardees
	Rajitha Senaratne, Minister of Health, the Democratic Socialist Republic of Sri Lanka Marisol Touraine, Minister of Social Affairs and Health, France* Omar Sey, Minister of Health and Social Welfare, the Gambia Rui Maria de Araújo, Prime Minister of the Democratic Republic of Timor-Leste Piyasakol Sakolsatayadhorn, Minister of Public Health, Kingdom of Thailand

*Source:*http://www.who.int/tobacco/wntd/awards/en/
*Director-General Special awards.

Globalization of marketing and trade also offers unprecedented opportunities for multinational companies to promote processed food and fast food high in fat, especially saturated and trans fats, salt and sugars. Processed foods include baby food, bakery products, canned/preserved food, chilled/frozen/dried processed food, confectionery, dairy, ice cream, noodles, oils and fats, pasta, ready meals, sauces, dressings and condiments, snack bars, soup, spreads, and sweet and savoury snacks. The packaged food market is huge. It is more than twice the size of the fruit and vegetable market in Mexico and the United States, and more than three times the size in the United Kingdom. This suggests a larger contribution of packaged foods than fresh foods to the diet in these countries, thus exposing people to diets high in fat, salt and sugar. In 2012, in the United States alone, the total advertising budget of fast food companies reached US$ 4.6 billion [13], giving an indication of the profitability of this sector. To put that amount in perspective, consider WHO, the world's leading public health agency that works tirelessly to promote and protect public health worldwide, with a total programme budget for 2016 and 2017 of only US$ 4.4 billion [14]. Out of that, a mere US$ 339.9 million was allocated to fight stroke, heart disease, diabetes, cancer, chronic respiratory diseases and other NCDs.

3. WHAT ARE THE TACTICS USED BY INDUSTRY TO UNDERMINE GOVERNMENT POLICIES TO PREVENT STROKE?

Tobacco, alcohol and processed food companies resort to devious tactics to undermine effective policy development and implementation in order to protect their profit margins [8 - 12, 15, 16].

They include:

- political lobbying and donations for public health initiatives;
- exaggerating the industries' economic importance;
- promoting ineffective measures such as self-regulation;
- manipulating and debating the scientific evidence;
- questioning the credibility of independent researchers;
- questioning the effectiveness of statutory regulation;

- creating strong and diverse opposing groups;
- undermining community concerns;
- framing unhealthy consumption behaviour as a personal responsibility issue;
- highlighting industry responsibility through highly publicized corporate social responsibility activities;
- industry funding of, and influence over, academic research;
- branding and mocking government regulatory control as "nanny state" policies;
- highlighting the importance of consumer choice even to health damaging products;
- creating brand awareness, including through sponsorship of sports and educational activities;
- portraying the industries as "part of the solution" to preventing the diseases caused by their products; and
- employing corporate social responsibility strategies as a means of shaping political environments and informing public perceptions.

The strategies of transnational tobacco corporations to undermine effective tobacco control policy has been widely documented. As a result, formal measures to exclude the industry from policy-making have been adopted in the WHO Framework Convention on Tobacco Control [17]. In contrast to the tobacco industry, alcohol and food industries are subject to less stringent forms of regulation. Consequently, these industries with vested interests in policy work often continue to play a central role in policy-making in many countries. Despite some important differences, the many similarities that exist between tobacco, alcohol and food industries in terms of market structure and political strategy do not justify the relatively weak regulatory approach taken towards alcohol and food industries [15, 16].

On the positive side, 10 major multinational food and beverage companies working through the International Food and Beverage Alliance (IFBA) have made pledges to support public health. These top 10 packaged food companies and soft drink companies account for 15% and 52%, respectively, of sales worldwide [17]. The pledges include initiatives to improve the nutrition quality of products and how these products are advertised to children. The litmus test would be to demonstrate the impact of implementing these commitments through independent audit and monitoring.

4. DO CHILDREN AND OTHER VULNERABLE GROUPS NEED PROTECTION FROM STROKE (NCDS)?

As the line between entertainment and advertising is increasingly blurred, industries target children and other vulnerable groups in a multitude of ways including:

- advertising on television and other media
- the internet
- social media
- viral marketing
- celebrity endorsements
- product placement in films
- competitions
- supermarket promotions and discounts, and
- smartphone games.

It is the moral responsibility of governments and all stakeholders to act on behalf of children to protect their health. NCDs manifest in adults, but the process that leads to these deadly diseases has its origin in childhood, when unhealthy consumption behaviours are adopted by children. Therefore, government efforts to prevent them must begin with children. Given the enormous potential harm to childrens' health, states have a duty to take all legislative and regulatory actions to protect children from exposure to tobacco, alcohol and unhealthy food.

People living in poverty and with lower levels of education are also more likely to be exposed to tobacco, alcohol and unhealthy diets and to develop stroke (NCDs). A social gradient is observed in tobacco use, with the rates of tobacco use decreasing with increasing socioeconomic status [18]. Similarly, a social gradient exists in risk from alcohol use [18]. Overweight and obesity have also become increasingly more prevalent among socially disadvantaged groups, particularly in high-income countries and urban areas of middle-income countries [19].

Strategies to prevent and control these diseases should, therefore, go hand in hand with an understanding of how their impact might potentially be distributed among the population, given that some groups would probably benefit more than others. As a minimum, it is important to ensure that interventions to address these diseases do not exacerbate existing inequities by benefiting those in the higher socioeconomic groups more than other groups of the population. Government action on social determinants of health and primary health care needs to be central in national health and NCD agendas.

5. ARE GOVERNMENTS DOING ENOUGH TO PREVENT CHILDHOOD OBESITY?

Obesity is a harbinger of diabetes, stroke and heart attacks. The frightening statistics on childhood obesity demonstrate how vulnerable children are to exposure to obesogenic environments that promote unhealthy diets and insufficient physical activity. According to WHO, currently, 42 million children under 5 are overweight or obese, an increase of about 11 million during the past

15 years. Almost half (48%) of these children live in Asia and 25% in Africa. In 2014, more than one in three (39%) adults worldwide aged 18 or older were overweight. Worldwide prevalence of obesity more than doubled between 1980 and 2014, with 11% of men and 15% of women (more than half a billion adults) being classified as obese [18].

Despite these alarming figures, only about 50 countries have a policy to reduce the impact on children of the marketing of foods and non-alcoholic beverages high in saturated fats, trans-fatty acids, free sugars or salt [2]. Only 6% of countries in the WHO African Region have a marketing policy in place. Marketing policies are particularly infrequent in low-income countries. Even though many countries are on the verge of a childhood obesity epidemic, only 18% of countries tax sugar-sweetened beverages, 7% have taxation incentives to promote physical activity and 8% tax foods high in fat, sugar or salt. Price subsidies for healthy foods are relatively low globally (21% of countries in the Region of the Americas and 10% or less of countries in other WHO regions) [1].

What needs to be done to curb obesity is clearly laid out in several seminal reports [19 - 21]. Regrettably, even developed countries are not taking robust, decisive, multisectoral actions required to address childhood obesity, even though they have the means to do so. The Government of the United Kingdom Childhood Obesity Plan, released recently, is a case in point [22]. One third of British children aged 2–15 years are overweight or obese. Already, the United Kingdom spends more on the treatment of obesity and diabetes than it does on the police, judiciary and fire service, put together [22]. Reducing obesity would safeguard health and save money. Yet, the Childhood Obesity Plan is far too weak to be effective. The plan aims to reduce childhood obesity by "encouraging" industry to cut the amount of sugar in food and drinks and primary school children to eat more healthily and stay active. Polices that are known to work have been jettisoned from the plan. There are no regulations to ban promotion of unhealthy food in supermarkets or advertising of junk food through television and social media. Producers and importers of soft drinks have been given two years to lower the sugar in their drinks. There are no binding targets or a monitoring framework. Over all, it appears that the interests of the food industry have been well taken care of at the cost of the health of British children.

As discussed above, tobacco, alcohol, processed and fast food industries are highly profitable and it is not in the industries' financial interest to cooperate with public health initiatives. However, when governments mandate regulations and legislate, these industries are compelled to fall in line. In the past, governments have legislated to make changes that are good for public health, such as wearing seat belts in vehicles, resulting in enormous public health benefit. Even though it may be politically unpalatable, governments need to take a similar approach to prevent stroke (NCDs), including childhood obesity.

6. WHAT ARE THE CHALLENGES THAT SLOW DOWN PREVENTION AND CONTROL OF STROKE (NCDS)?

In addition to powerful forces that drive the stroke burden mentioned above, many other challenges persist that slow down action to combat stroke (NCDs). These include:

• NCDs lower priority;
• unstable funding flows for health and NCDs that hamper health sector planning;
• poor coordination between ministries of health and finance;
• low revenue generation through taxation;
• inadequate capacity to actually spend the money set aside for health;
• lack of priority given to prevention and primary health care;
• lack of collaboration between health and other ministries resulting in weak multisectoral action;
• viewing NCDs as "health issues" and "single disease" entities;
• lack of adequate infrastructure;
• human resource constraints;
• inadequate capacity to participate in international rule-making and the negotiation process for healthy trade and marketing practices; and
• weak institutions resulting in weak policy and regulatory environments and lack of monitoring of implementation of existing policies.

Among these multiple challenges, lack of sustainable domestic and international financing is by far the most important barrier [21, 23 - 25]. For national NCD action to be implemented and sustained, any new financing will have to depend primarily on domestic public resources. International financing needs to complement domestic financing mainly through strengthening institutional capacity to fight NCDs. Despite the inclusion of NCDs in the Sustainable Development Goals, the main focus of international financing will continue to be on combating communicable diseases. In 2010, the *World health report* estimated that low-income countries would need to spend, on average, around US$ 60 per person by 2015 to deliver priority health interventions [25]. Further analysis in 2015 updated these estimates to US$ 86 per person, highlighting that countries would find it difficult to get close to universal health coverage if public spending on health is less than 4–5% of GDP. In 2014, per person expenditure on health in 44 countries was less than US$ 86 (Table **2.2**).

Table 2.2. Health expenditure per capita by country for 2014.

Per capita total expenditure on health at average exchange rate (US$)	Countries*
<86	Afghanistan, Bangladesh, Benin, Burkina Faso, Burundi, Central African Republic, Cambodia, Cameroon, Chad, Democratic Republic of the Congo, Eritrea, Ethiopia, Gambia, Comoros, Côte d'Ivoire, Ghana, Guinea, Guinea-Bissau, Haiti, India, Kenya, Kyrgyzstan Lao People's Democratic Republic, Liberia, Madagascar, Malawi, Mali, Mauritania, Mozambique, Myanmar, Nepal, Pakistan, Niger, Rwanda, Senegal, Sierra Leone, Syrian Arab Republic, Tajikistan, Timor-Leste, Togo, Uganda, United Republic of Tanzania, Yemen, Zambia
86 to <500	Albania, Algeria, Angola, Armenia, Azerbaijan, Belarus, Bhutan, Bolivia, Bosnia and Herzegovina, Botswana, Cabo Verde, China, Congo, Djibouti, Dominica, Dominican Republic, Egypt, El Salvador, Fiji, Gabon, Georgia, Guatemala, Guyana, Honduras, Indonesia, Iran (Islamic Republic of), Iraq, Jamaica, Jordan, Kiribati, Lesotho, Libya, Malaysia, Mauritius Micronesia, Mongolia, Montenegro, Morocco, Namibia, Nicaragua, Nigeria, Papua New Guinea, Paraguay, Peru, Philippines, Republic of Moldova, Saint Lucia, Samoa, San Marino, Sao Tome and Principe, Seychelles, Solomon Islands, Sri Lanka, Sudan, Swaziland, Thailand, The former Yugoslav Republic of Macedonia, Tonga, Tunisia, Turkmenistan, Ukraine, Uzbekistan, Vanuatu, Viet Nam
500 to <1000	Antigua and Barbuda, Argentina, Brazil, Brunei Darussalam, Bulgaria, Colombia, Cook Islands, Cuba, Costa Rica, Ecuador, Equatorial Guinea, Grenada, Kazakhstan, Latvia, Lebanon, Marshall Islands, Mexico, Nauru, Oman, Panama, Poland, Romania, Russian Federation, Saint Kitts and Nevis, Saint Vincent and the Grenadines, Serbia, South Africa, Suriname, Turkey, Tuvalu, Venezuela (Bolivarian Republic of)
1000 to <2000	Bahrain, Bahamas, Barbados, Chile, Croatia, Cyprus, Czech Republic, Estonia, Greece, Hungary, Kuwait, Lithuania, Maldives, Niue, Palau, Saudi Arabia, Slovakia, Trinidad and Tobago, United Arab Emirates, Uruguay
2000 to <3000	Israel, Malta, Portugal, Qatar, Republic of Korea, Singapore, Slovenia, Spain
3000 to <4000	Andorra, Italy, Japan, United Kingdom of Great Britain and Northern Ireland
4000 to <5000	Belgium, Finland, France, Iceland, Ireland, New Zealand
5000 to <6000	Austria, Canada, Germany, Netherlands
6000 to <8000	Australia, Denmark, Sweden
8000 to 10 000	Luxembourg, Monaco, Norway. Monaco, Switzerland, United States of America

* Data not available for Democratic People's Republic of Korea, Somalia, South Sudan and Zimbabwe.
Source: World Health Organization Global Health Observatory data 2016 http://apps.who.int/gho/data/view.main.HEALTHEXPCAPAFG?lang=en).

The per person income is many fold higher in high-income countries compared to developing countries. For example, while the United States spends US$ 9402 per person, a developing country such as Rwanda only spends US$ 52 per person for health. Thus, interventions and vertical programme approaches that are used to tackle stroke (NCDs) in high-income countries should not be exported to developing countries using external aid. These approaches are neither affordable nor sustainable for developing countries and worsen existing inequities. The main focus of developing countries should be on implementing very cost-effective interventions (WHO best buys) to tackle stroke (NCDs). These include preventing first and recurrent attacks of strokes by providing treatment to high risk people through a primary health care approach [31]. Establishing affordable stroke unit care should also receive due consideration at least in medium resource settings (see Chapters 4 and 5).

Increasing domestic resource mobilization to finance NCDs is a challenge for many low- and middle-income countries with competing health priorities. However, not financing national NCD efforts is not a viable option for any country. In the event of inaction against NCDs the cumulative losses in the national product of low- and middle-income countries for the period 2011–2025 has been estimated at more than US$ 7 trillion [26].

7. IS GOVERNMENT ACTION MATCHING THE SIZE AND COMPLEXITY OF THE STROKE (NCDS) BURDEN?

Most high-income countries have made progress in addressing stroke (NCDs). In the majority of low- and middle-income countries action is not matching the size and complexity of the burden. In some there is frightening inaction [2]. Although multisectoral collaboration is fundamental to stroke (NCDs) prevention, about two thirds of countries still have not established a national multisectoral mechanism to oversee policy coherence and accountability of sectors beyond health. Only half (53%) of countries have an operational, multisectoral national action plan that integrates action across NCDs that share risk factors.

Even though sustainable funding of NCD activities is a major challenge, two thirds of countries do not use earmarked taxes on tobacco, alcohol or unhealthy food items to supplement the NCD budget. About 39% of countries also do not use insurance funds to support NCD-related activities. Even though NCDs require long-term investments, 63% of countries rely on international donors for NCD prevention and control. Despite the serious potential damage that tobacco and alcohol inflict on health, 13% of countries still do not have a tax on tobacco products and 20% of countries have no taxation on alcohol.

Although reducing salt intake to healthy levels is an effective intervention to prevent stroke, globally, only 38% of countries are implementing policies to reduce population salt consumption. None of the low-income countries have implemented policies to reduce population salt consumption and prevalence of these policies are also very low (13%) in lower-middle-income countries.

8. WHAT KIND OF COUNTRY ACTION IS ESSENTIAL FOR PREVENTION OF STROKE (NCDS)?

Stroke (NCDs) cannot be prevented by action within the health sector alone. Such action on its own will not be sustainable. A public health approach that combines prevention, treatment and monitoring in a balanced manner is required to tackle stroke (NCDs). All governments need to ensure that a national multisectoral plan is developed and implemented with active engagement of relevant sectors such as finance, agriculture and trade. The WHO 2013–2020 Global Action Plan for the Prevention and Control of NCDs (Global NCD Action Plan), identifies the strategic objectives (Table **2.3**) that need attention in any country embarking on an initiative to fight stroke (NCDs) [27]. As mentioned above, creating conducive environments to change consumption behaviour and strengthening health systems are two of these six strategic areas.

Table 2.3. Strategic objectives of the Global NCD Action Plan 2013–2020.

1. **Raise the priority** accorded to the prevention and control of NCDs in national agendas through strengthened international cooperation and advocacy.
2. **Strengthen national capacity, leadership, governance, multisectoral action and partnerships** to accelerate country response for the prevention and control of NCDs.
3. **Reduce modifiable risk factors for NCDs** and underlying social determinants through creation of health-promoting environments.
4. **Strengthen and orient health systems** to address NCDs and the underlying social determinants through people-centred primary health care and universal health coverage.
5. **Promote and support national capacity** for high-quality research and development for the prevention and control of NCDs.
6. **Monitor the trends and determinants of NCDs** and evaluate progress in their prevention and control.

Source: Global action plan for the prevention and control of non-communicable diseases 2013–2020. Geneva: World Health Organization; 2013.

In addition to the Framework Convention on Tobacco Control [17], several global frameworks and international agreements have been drawn up to provide the foundation and framework for country action (*e.g.* the Global NCD Action Plan 2013–2020) global strategy on reducing the harmful use of alcohol and global strategy on diet physical activity and health, with recommendations on the marketing of foods and non-alcoholic beverages to children and report on financing for universal health coverage [25, 28 - 30]. These provide the foundation for country action to create conducive environments and to strengthen health systems. Further, there are very cost-effective interventions known as best buys to address stroke (NCDs) (Table **2.4**) [31].

Table 2.4. Very cost-effective NCD interventions (best buys), affordable to all countries.

Tobacco
■ Reduce affordability of tobacco products by increasing tobacco excise taxes
■ Create by law completely smoke-free environments in all indoor workplaces, public places and public transport
■ Warn people of the dangers of tobacco and tobacco smoke through effective health warnings and mass media campaigns
■ Ban all forms of tobacco advertising, promotion and sponsorship

Harmful use of alcohol
■ Regulate commercial and public availability of alcohol
■ Restrict or ban alcohol advertising and promotions
■ Use pricing policies such as excise tax increases on alcoholic beverages

Diet and physical activity
■ Reduce salt intake
■ Replace trans fats with unsaturated fats
■ Implement public awareness programmes on diet and physical activity
■ Promote and protect breastfeeding

Cardiovascular disease and diabetes
■ Drug therapy (including glycaemic control for diabetes mellitus and control of hypertension using a total risk approach) and counselling to individuals who have had a heart attack or stroke and to persons with high risk ($\geq 30\%$) of a fatal and nonfatal cardiovascular event in the next 10 years
■ Acetylsalicylic acid (aspirin) for acute myocardial infarction

Cancer
■ Prevention of liver cancer through hepatitis B immunization
■ Prevention of cervical cancer through screening (visual inspection with acetic acid [*VIA*] linked with timely treatment of pre-cancerous lesions)

Source: Global action plan for the prevention and control of non-communicable diseases 2013–2020. Geneva: World Health Organization; 2013.

Banning all forms of tobacco advertising, restricting or banning alcohol advertising, promoting breast-feeding, implementing public awareness programmes on diet and physical activity, replacing trans fats with polyunsaturated fats, and preventing stroke and heart attacks by treatment of high-risk groups in primary care are very effective low-cost public health measures within the reach of all governments. Clearly, implementing these interventions require collaboration with other sectors such as finance, trade, media, education and others, even though the primary responsibility lies with the health sector.

Price and tax measures on tobacco, alcohol and unhealthy food can reduce unhealthy consumption patterns and health-care costs, as well as representing a revenue stream for financing national agendas on NCDs and the Sustainable Development Goals [24, 25]. To date, at least 30 countries are earmarking tobacco tax revenues for public health purposes. Thailand, for example, has used revenues generated from a 2% surtax on tobacco and alcohol to fund ThaiHealth, a state run health promotion foundation that supports health promotion activities [32]. In 2014, ThaiHealth, garnered the equivalent of US$ 125 million from the surcharge, and utilized the revenue for programming of activities to control tobacco and alcohol and for promotion of physical activity and healthy diet. In 2012, the Philippines passed the Sin Tax Reform bill that increased taxes on all tobacco and alcohol projects, providing a new injection of funding for its universal health coverage scheme [33]. In the first year of operation more than US$ 1.2 billion was raised that enabled expansion of coverage of basic health services to the poorest and vulnerable Filipinos. Such visionary action is highly commendable and worthy of emulation by policy-makers and politicians in other developing countries that have to grapple with the challenge of domestic health financing.

9. WHAT COULD GOVERNMENTS DO TO REDUCE EXPOSURE OF PEOPLE TO BEHAVIOURAL RISK FACTORS OF STROKE (NCDS)?

What, and how much, people eat, drink and smoke and how they expend energy depend on their socioeconomic, political, physical and cultural environments. To prevent stroke mere *encouragement* by governments is not adequate. Governments have the responsibility to *create* environments that support healthy behaviour. Supportive environments make healthy choices and behaviours easy, attractive and affordable and unhealthy choices and behaviours difficult, unattractive and unaffordable. This transformation of environments can be made only through regulatory and legislative policies. For example, by prohibiting advertising, banning the sale to children, increasing the price of tobacco and alcohol products, banning smoking in public places, a conducive environment is created for reducing the use of tobacco and alcohol. In addition, in some countries, fiscal tools have been applied to control tobacco and alcohol use. Governments have imposed special taxes on tobacco (Table **2.5**) and alcohol as raising taxes is the most effective way of reducing their use. In some of these countries, income derived from taxation on tobacco and alcohol is used to promote healthy behaviour. These bold measures have produced positive results for individuals and society, while at the same time generating income to improve the nation's health and well-being.

Table 2.5. Countries reporting taxation on tobacco products with at least 70% excise tax share in final consumer price.

High-income	Austria, Belgium, Canada, Chile, Croatia, Cyprus, Czech Republic, Denmark, Estonia, Finland, France, Germany, Greece, Ireland, Israel, Italy, Latvia, Lithuania, Luxembourg, Malta, Netherlands, New Zealand, Poland, Portugal, San Marino, Slovakia, Slovenia, Spain, United Kingdom of Great Britain and Northern Ireland

(Table 2.5) contd.....

Upper-middle income	Argentina, Bosnia and Herzegovina, Bulgaria, Costa Rica, Ecuador, Hungary, Jordan, Mauritius, Montenegro, Romania, Serbia, Seychelles, Niue, Thailand, The former Yugoslav Republic of Macedonia, Tonga, Tunisia, Turkey, Venezuela (Bolivarian Republic of Venezuela)
Lower-middle income	Egypt, Kiribati, Morocco, Philippines, Sri Lanka, Sudan, Ukraine
Low-income	Bangladesh, Madagascar, Tajikistan, West Bank and Gaza Strip

Source: WHO report on the global tobacco epidemic 2015. Geneva: World Health Organization; 2015.

Similarly, to promote a healthy diet a conducive environment needs to be created using legislative and regulatory measures. Such measures should aim to reduce the level of salt added to food, increase availability and affordability of fruit and vegetables, reduce saturated fatty acids in food and replace them with unsaturated fatty acids, reduce the content of sugars in food and non-alcoholic beverages to limit excess energy (calorie) intake and reduce portion size and energy density of foods. For example, fiscal policies that lead to at least a 20% increase in the retail price of sugary drinks would result in proportional reductions in consumption of such products [34]. Lower consumption of sugar in turn can reduce obesity, type 2 diabetes and tooth decay. It is simply unrealistic to expect that these changes will happen through self-regulation of the food industry.

Policy measures also need to be implemented in cooperation with other sectors such as education, youth affairs and sports to promote physical activity through activities of daily living. These policy measures could include urban planning and transport policies to improve the accessibility and safety of, and supportive infrastructure for, walking and cycling, creation of built and natural environments that support physical activity in different settings, including schools, workplaces, hospitals and in the wider community.

The above measures, including legislative and regulatory actions, can be spearheaded only by governments, ministers and ministries. The Minister and Ministry of Health often need to guide the action in collaboration with Ministers and Ministries of Finance, Agriculture, Transport, Trade and others. Primary concerns of these ministries, however, are not really focused on health. Therefore, not surprisingly collaboration between ministries to promote good health is rare. It becomes a reality mainly in countries in which presidents and/or prime ministers oversee and drive the inter-ministerial collaboration with fiscal and programmatic incentives. Governance tools that allow the central government to promote multisectoral collaboration and policy coherence for health and well-being of the population include structures (*e.g.* committees dedicated to collaboration), processes (*e.g.* joint planning and evaluation), financial frameworks (*e.g.* fiscal mechanisms fostering intersectoral activities) and mandates (*e.g.* laws or regulations imposing accountability).

There needs to be heightened awareness and knowledge of policy-makers and politicians, as well as that of the public, of the role and actions of industry and of their conflicts of interest with public health. Research on corporate social responsibility practices and marketing campaigns could provide a strong evidence base regarding industry tactics and influence. The formation of national public health coalitions could help to strengthen advocacy initiatives against unhealthy consumption behaviours. Stronger collaboration is required between ministries of health, nongovernmental organizations, independent academics and researchers [35]. Media can play a vital role to effectively shift perceptions of harm from unhealthy consumption behaviour away from the individual and towards the unhealthy commodity. Nongovernmental organizations have the important role of a watchdog to blunt industries' efforts to undermine public health policies.

10. HOW CAN HEALTH SYSTEMS BE STRENGTHENED FOR COST-EFFECTIVE PREVENTION AND CONTROL OF STROKE (NCDS)?

Health systems need to be transformed to address stroke cost effectively. Stroke care that is focused on high technology inpatient care alone will neither fully protect against financial risk nor cover services that improve health cost effectively. It requires a public health approach, as discussed above, including strengthening of primary health care. Due to financial and human resource constraints, governments of many low- and middle-income countries are unlikely to be able to provide most of the advanced treatment for acute stroke that is freely available in public sector health facilities (see Chapter 4). In a recent global capacity assessment survey, countries from the low-income and lower-middl--income in the WHO African Region and the Region of the Americas groupings reported provision for stroke care in less than 25% of public sector health facilities [2]. Strokes can be prevented cost effectively if high-risk individuals are detected early in primary care and managed [6]. Those at high risk include those with hypertension, diabetes, other cardiovascular risk factors and a past history of stroke or heart disease. This is a very cost-effective intervention that should be available in all primary health care facilities [36]. It should be part of the basic services package in all universal health coverage schemes.

Currently, there are major gaps in access to basic technologies and medicines that prevent the implementation of this very effective primary care intervention. According to the most recent global capacity assessment survey [2], people do not have access to blood glucose measurement in primary care in 15% of countries. About one third of the countries do not have urine strips for glucose and albumin measurement. There were major gaps in access to essential medicines for stroke prevention and metformin was generally not available in 18% of countries, angiotensin converting enzyme inhibitors in 21%, beta-blockers in 22%, calcium channel blockers in 24%, insulin in 18%, sulfonylurea in 31% and statins in 37%.

More detailed studies reveal more critical gaps in the provision of basic technologies and medicines in primary care in low- and middle-income countries [37]. Context-specific strategies will be required to address multiple gaps in health systems related to financing, access to basic technologies and medicines, the health workforce, service delivery and quality, and health information and referral, particularly at the primary care level. Managing acute stroke in developing country settings with no access to CT scanners and stroke units, require pragmatic approaches. They include the judicious use of aspirin and proven supportive care measures such as maintaining normal blood sugar and body temperature, prompt treatment of fits, prevention of aspiration and blood clots in leg veins and early mobilization. Stroke units have been shown to improve morbidity, mortality and other outcomes of stroke. Efforts need to be made to establish low-cost organized care (stroke units) linking them to existing medical wards in hospitals and primary care.

11. DOES THE GLOBAL HEALTH AND DEVELOPMENT MILIEU SUPPORT THE ACTION OF GOVERNMENTS?

The global health and development environment has never been more supportive of government action to prevent stroke (NCDs). In 2011, at the United Nations High-level Meeting on Non-communicable Diseases, heads of state and government formally recognized NCDs as a major threat to economies and societies and placed them high on the global health and development agenda [38]. They agreed on a wide-ranging set of commitments to address the global burden of NCDs. WHO was assigned a leadership and coordination role in supporting national efforts to meet these commitments. Three years later, ministers of health of 194 WHO Member States endorsed the Global NCD Action Plan 2013–2020 with nine concrete global targets [27] (Table **2.6**).

The action plan is meant to be implemented collectively by Member States, international partners and WHO. In July 2013, the United Nations Secretary-General established the United Nations Interagency Task Force on NCDs to facilitate the response of the United Nations system to national demands for support for multisectoral action. This task force reports to the Economic and Social Council (ECOSOC) through the Secretary-General [39]. In May 2014, the WHO Global Coordination Mechanism on NCDs was established in particular to facilitate contributions from non-state actors [40].

Table 2.6. Global voluntary targets for prevention and control of NCDs.

In May 2013, the Sixty-sixth World Health Assembly adopted the comprehensive global monitoring framework for the prevention and control of NCDs. This framework includes 25 indicators to monitor trends and assess progress made in the prevention and control of NCDs; nine areas were selected from the 25 indicators to be targets. All targets were set for 2025, with a baseline of 2010. The global voluntary targets are:

Target 1. A 25% relative reduction in the risk of premature mortality from CVD, cancer, diabetes or CRD.

Target 2. At least 10% relative reduction in the harmful use of alcohol.

Target 3. A 10% relative reduction in prevalence of insufficient physical activity.

Target 4. A 30% relative reduction in mean population intake of salt/sodium.

Target 5. A 30% relative reduction in prevalence of current tobacco use.

Target 6. A 25% relative reduction in the prevalence of raised blood pressure.

Target 7. Halt the rise in diabetes and obesity.

Target 8. At least 50% of eligible people receive drug therapy and counselling (including glycaemic control) to prevent heart attacks and strokes.

Target 9. An 80% availability of the affordable basic technologies and essential medicines, including generics, required to treat major NCDs in both public and private facilities.

The first global voluntary target is closely linked to SDG Target 3.4, to reduce premature NCD mortality by one third by 2030.

CRD = chronic respiratory disease
CVD = cardiovascular disease
Source: Global action plan for the prevention and control of noncommunicable diseases 2013–2020. Geneva: World Health Organization; 2013.

More recently, in September 2015, the United Nations General Assembly formally adopted the 2030 Agenda for Sustainable Development, along with 17 Sustainable Development Goals and targets [41]. The goals address global priorities, including ending poverty and hunger, reducing social inequality, achieving good health and well-being, tackling climate change and preserving the Earth's natural resources (see Chapter 6). Six targets of the 2030 Agenda for Sustainable Development are related to NCDs: a one third reduction in premature mortality from NCDs by 2030; improvements in tobacco control; reducing substance abuse, including harmful use of alcohol; supporting research and development of vaccines and medicines for NCDs that primarily affect developing countries, as well as providing access to affordable essential medicines and vaccines for NCDs; reducing deaths and illnesses related to hazardous chemicals, as well as air, water and soil pollution and contamination and on universal health coverage.

12. SHOULD GOVERNMENTS BE HELD ACCOUNTABLE FOR INACTION?

Governments are the custodians of the health of people and are accountable for taking action to safeguard their health. To reverse the stroke (NCDs) epidemic, a different world order is required that can hold governments accountable for the health of people. However, key ingredients required to bring about policy change to combat stroke (NCDs) are already in place at the global level. First, commitments have been made by the heads of state and governments to accelerate action to address NCDs [36]. Second, policies and interventions affordable to all countries have been identified [20, 21, 27]. Third, there is an agreement on what should be done and how it is to be done [31, 36]. What is now required is implementation at the country level. In other words, governments need to deliver on their commitments.

There is a global accountability framework in place for reporting on progress on prevention and control of NCDs. WHO has been mandated to report on progress of addressing NCDs to the World Health Assembly, the United Nations General Assembly and the United Nations Economic and Social Council. With regard to reporting to the World Health Assembly, the WHO Director-General will submit reports on progress made in implementing the Global NCD Action Plan 2013–2020 to the World Health Assembly in 2016, 2018 and 2021. A WHO report on the progress achieved in NCD prevention and control will also be submitted to the United Nations General Assembly by the end of 2017.

Data are vital to operationalize any accountability framework. In this context, it is of concern that there are at least 21 countries without a system for routine collection of information on the number and causes of death. In addition, around 42 countries have not conducted any recent (*i.e.* in 2010 or later) national adult risk factor surveys [2]. The global voluntary targets and indicators provide a sound framework for global monitoring and for benchmarking the performance of countries. However, global monitoring alone will not be sufficient. A collective international response will be required to assist countries that have been left behind. At the national level, policy-makers, politicians, academia and civil society will need to independently review the monitoring results and take remedial action to accelerate progress in NCD prevention and control.

CONCLUDING REMARKS

A multisectoral policy framework involving ministries of health, finance, trade, agriculture and others is required to prevent stroke (NCDs). Supportive policy environments make healthy choices and behaviours easy, and unhealthy choices and behaviours difficult. To address stroke and other NCDs, countries need to strengthen their ability to overcome barriers driven by power, profits and politics. Civil society can play a vital role in ensuring that governments, ministries and ministers are held accountable for action to address NCDs to the people they are designed to serve. Regrettably, in many countries, people have no voice and civil society has neither the capacity nor the freedom to hold governments accountable for their actions. As discussed in Chapter 3, low-and middle-income countries carry the major share of the global stroke burden. New developments and scientific advances discussed in Chapters 4 and 5 will have a significant impact on the global stroke burden, but only if they are implemented both in rich and poor countries.

CONFLICT OF INTEREST

The author declares no conflict of interest, financial or otherwise.

ACKNOWLEDGEMENTS

Ms AvisAnne Julien is thanked for copy-editing.

REFERENCES

[1]   Preventing tobacco use among youth and young adults. A report of the surgeon general

[2]   Noncommunicable diseases progress monitor. 2015. Available at: http://apps.who.int/iris/bitstream/ 10665/184688/1/9789241509459_eng.pdf?ua=1

[3]   WHO Report on the global tobacco epidemic 2015. 2015. Available at: http://www.who.int/ tobacco/global_report/2015/en/

[4]   WHO framework convention on tobacco control. 2016. Available at: http://www.who.int/fctc/ mediacentre/news/2016/legal-victories-against-tobacco-industry/en/

[5]   WHO framework convention on tobacco control. 2016. Available at: http://www.who.int/fctc/ mediacentre/news/2016/international-tribunal-states-rights-to-protect-health-through-t/en/

[6]   Australia wins international legal battle with Philip Morris over plain packaging. The Guardian Available at: https://www.theguardian.com/australia-news/2015/dec/18/australia-wins-internatio-al-legal-battle-with-philip-morris-over-plain-packaging

[7]   Marketing and alcohol fact sheet 2013. Institute of Alcohol Studies: London 2013. Available at: http://www.ias.org.uk/uploads/pdf/Factsheets/Marketing%20and%20alcohol%20FS%20May%202013 .pdf

[8]   Moodie R, Stuckler D, Monteiro C, *et al*. Profits and pandemics: prevention of harmful effects of tobacco, alcohol, and ultra-processed food and drink industries. Lancet 2013; 381(9867): 670-9. [http://dx.doi.org/10.1016/S0140-6736(12)62089-3] [PMID: 23410611]

[9]   Avery MR, Droste N, Giorgi C, *et al*. Mechanisms of influence: Alcohol industry submissions to the inquiry into fetal alcohol spectrum disorders. Drug Alcohol Rev 2016; 35(6): 665-72. [http://dx.doi.org/10.1111/dar.12399] [PMID: 27246440]

[10]   Savell E, Fooks G, Gilmore AB. How does the alcohol industry attempt to influence marketing regulations? A systematic review. Addiction 2016; 111(1): 18-32. [http://dx.doi.org/10.1111/add.13048] [PMID: 26173765]

[11]   Paukštė E, Liutkutė V, Stelemėkas M, Goštautaitė Midttun N, Veryga A. Overturn of the proposed alcohol advertising ban in Lithuania. Addiction 2014; 109(5): 711-9. [http://dx.doi.org/10.1111/add.12495] [PMID: 24588798]

[12]   Zhang C, Monteiro M. Tactics and practices of the alcohol industry in Latin America: What can policy makers do? Int J Alcohol Drug Res 2013; 2(2): 75-86.

[13]   Yale Rudd Center for Food policy and obesity. Fast food ranking marketing tables 2012–2013 Available at: http://www.fastfoodmarketing.org/media/fastfoodfacts_marketingrankings.pdf

[14]   World Health Organization programme budget 2016–2017 Available at: http://www.who.int/ about/finances-accountability/budget/PB201617_en.pdf

[15]   Smith K, Dorfman L, Freudenberg N, *et al.* Tobacco, alcohol, and processed food industries: Why do public health practitioners view them so differently? Front Public Health 2016; 4: 64. [http://dx.doi.org/10.3389/fpubh.2016.00064] [PMID: 27148511]

[16]   Hawkins B, Holden C, Eckhardt J, Lee K. Reassessing policy paradigms: a comparison of the global tobacco and alcohol industries. Glob Pub Health 2016; 1.19. [http://dx.doi.org/10.1080/17441692.2016.1161815]

[17]   WHO framework convention on tobacco control 2003. Available at: http://whqlibdoc.who. int/publications/2003/9241591013.pdf

[18]   Equity, social determinants and public health programmes 2010. Available at: http://apps.who. int/iris/bitstream/10665/44289/1/9789241563970_eng.pdf

[19]   Report of the commission on ending childhood obesity. Geneva: World Health Organization 2016.

[20]   Global status report on noncommunicable diseases 2010 2011. Available at: http://www.who. int/nmh/publications/ncd_report_full_en.pdf

[21]   Global status report on noncommunicable diseases 2014. Geneva: World Health Organization 2014.

[22]   Government HM. Childhood obesity; a plan for action 2016. Available at: https://www.gov.uk/ government/uploads/system/uploads/attachment_data/file/546588/Childhood_obesity_2016__2__acc. pdf

[23]   Public financing for health in Africa; from Abuja to the SDGs. Geneva: World Health Organization 2016.

[24]   Addis Ababa action agenda, a new framework to finance the SDGs. New York: United Nations 2015.

[25]   World health report 2010 Financing for universal health coverage. Geneva: World Health Organization 2010.

[26]   From burden to "Best Buys": reducing the economic impact of noncommunicable diseases in low- and middle- income countries. Geneva: World Economic Forum 2011.

[27]   Global action plan for the prevention and control of noncommunicable diseases 2013–2020 2013. Available at: http://apps.who.int/iris/

[28]   Resolution WHA57. Global strategy on diet, physical activity and health 2004. Available at: http://apps.who.int/gb/ebwha/pdf_files/WHA57/A57_R17-en.pdf

[29]   Resolution WHA63. Global strategy to reduce the harmful use of alcohol. Sixty-third World Health Assembly, Geneva 2010. Available at: http://apps.who.int/gb/ebwha/pdf_files/ WHA63/A63_R13-en.pdf

[30]   A framework for implementing the set of recommendations on the marketing of foods and non-alcoholic beverages to children. Geneva: World Health Organization 2012.

[31]   Scaling up action against noncommunicable diseases: How much will it cost? 2011. Available at: http://www.who.int/nmh/publications/cost_of_inaction/en/

[32]   Thai health promotion foundation. Available at: http://en.thaihealth.or.th

[33]   Tax S. Official gazette of the republic of Philippines Available at: http://www.gov.ph/sin-tax/

[34]   Fiscal policies for diet and the prevention of noncommunicable diseases. Geneva: World Health Organization 2016.

[35]   Mendis S, Norrving B, Davis S. World Health Organization working with the World Stroke Organization/Civil Society in the combat of stroke. Stroke 2014; 45(10): e206-7. [Epub 2 September 2014].

[http://dx.doi.org/10.1161/STROKEAHA.114.005446] [PMID: 25184358]

[36]   Package of essential noncommunicable disease interventions (WHO PEN) for primary health care in low-resource settings. 2010. Available at: http://www.who.int/nmh/publications/essential_ncd_interventions_lr_settings.pdf

[37]   Mendis S, Al Bashir I, Dissanayake L, *et al.* Gaps in capacity in primary care in low-resource settings for implementation of essential noncommunicable disease interventions. Int J Hypertens 2012; 2012: 584041.
[http://dx.doi.org/10.1155/2012/584041] [PMID: 23251789]

[38]   Resolution 66/2. Political declaration of the high-level meeting of the general assembly on the prevention and control of non-communicable diseases. Sixty-sixth session of the United Nations General Assembly New York: United Nations 2011.

[39]   United Nations economic and social council document E/2013/L23 United Nations interagency task Force on the prevention and control of noncommunicable diseases Geneva: United Nations Available at: http://www.who.int/nmh/events/2013/E.2013.L.23_tobacco.pdf

[40]   Provisional agenda item131 Prevention and control of noncommunicable diseases Terms of reference for the global coordination mechanism on the prevention and control of noncommunicable diseases. Geneva: Sixty-seventh World Health Assembly 2014.

[41]   Resolution A/RES/70/1. Transforming our world: the 2030 Agenda for Sustainable Development. Adopted by the United Nations General Assembly, New York 2015. Available at: http://www.un.org/ga/search/view_doc.asp?symbol=A/RES/70/1&Lang=E

CHAPTER 3

Global Stroke Burden and Stroke Prevention

Rita V. Krishnamurthi[1,*], **Priya Parmar**[1], **Graeme J. Hankey**[2] and **Valery L. Feigin**[1]

[1] National Institute for Stroke and Applied Neurosciences, Auckland University of Technology, Auckland, New Zealand

[2] School of Medicine and Pharmacology, The University of Western Australia, Department of Neurology, Sir Charles Gairdner Hospital, Perth, Australia Western Australian Neuroscience Research Institute (WANRI), Perth, Australia

Abstract: Population ageing and increasing exposure to behavioural and environmental risk factors are increasing the worldwide burden of stroke. Since 1990, there has been a significant increase in absolute numbers of strokes and the number of deaths from stroke. The burden of stroke is higher in low- and middle-income countries and, in particular, increasing in the younger age groups. The major risk factors for stroke are well established, and many of these, particularly behavioural risk factors such as tobacco use, harmful use of alcohol, unhealthy diet and physical inactivity, are modifiable. Hence, stroke is a highly preventable disease. Primary prevention is the key strategy for reducing the global health impact of stroke. This chapter presents the most recent updates from the Global Burden of Diseases, Injuries and Risk Factors Study (GBD) 2013 studies and discusses stroke prevention strategies.

Keywords: Carotid artery stenting, Carotid endarterectomy, DALYs, Epidemiology, Global Burden of Diseases, Global burden, Incidence, Injuries and Risk Factors Study (GBD), Low- and middle-income countries prevention, Mobile technology, Mortality, Prevalence, Stroke.

INTRODUCTION

This chapter addresses the following questions.

1. What is the current global disease pattern (epidemiology) of stroke?
2. Are there differences in low- and middle-income countries compared to high-income countries?
3. Are there differences in sex in stroke burden?
4. Why should stroke prevention be a priority?

* **Corresponding author Rita V. Krishnamurthi:** National Institute for Stroke and Applied Neurosciences, Auckland University of Technology, Auckland, New Zealand; Tel: +649 921 9999; Fax: +649 921 9260; E-mail: rkrishna@aut.ac.nz

5. What are the current stroke prevention strategies?
6. What are the gaps in stroke prevention strategies and how can they be addressed?
7. What are the current surgical stroke prevention strategies?
8. What are the future directions in surgical prevention of stroke?

1. WHAT IS THE CURRENT GLOBAL DISEASE PATTERN (EPIDEMIOLOGY) OF STROKE?

The global impact of stroke is significant and rising. Stroke is the second major cause of death and the third leading cause of disability worldwide [1]. Its impact is felt on many levels; along with deleterious health-related consequences; stroke also has a major social, psychological and economic impact on the patients, their families and society [2]. The absolute numbers of strokes and the prevalence (the number of cases per 100 000 people studied) of stroke are projected to rise due to the ageing population of the world and exposure to risk factors. Due to the enormity of its impact, estimating and tracking its burden over time in terms of stroke incidence (rate of occurrence of new cases of stroke), prevalence, disability-adjusted life years (DALYs, a metric to describe years of healthy life lost) and mortality (death rate) worldwide and within countries and regions are eminently important. For example, if DALYs (in the context of stroke) for an individual equal to 10, it means that the individual lost 10 years of life free of disabilities due to stroke. Population wise, if DALYs equal to 100,000, it means that 100 000 years of life free of disabilities are lost due to stroke. Given that stroke is a heterogeneous disorder, it is also important to study the epidemiology of stroke by its subtypes – ischaemic stroke (due to the blockage of an artery supplying blood to the brain) and haemorrhagic stroke (due to the intracranial rupture of an artery supplying blood to the brain) – as the risk factors and outcomes of these two types of stroke may vary. Accurate and up-to-date estimates that also identify disparities in burden by countries and regions, race/ethnicity and sex allow health-care planning by governments and health ministries to allocate resources and manage the current and projected future burden. Importantly, stroke is a highly preventable disease by way of the adequate control of modifiable risk factors. The most effective way to reduce the impact of stroke is to prevent its occurrence in the first place (primary prevention) [3]. Therefore, identifying the prevalence and impact of modifiable risk factors (*e.g.* tobacco use, harmful use of alcohol, unhealthy diet and physical inactivity) is crucial for informing and planning the implementation of both current and novel prevention strategies.

Well-designed population-based epidemiological studies provide the most reliable source of information on current trends in stroke incidence, prevalence, DALYs and mortality [4]. In countries that are resource poor, population-based stroke incidence studies may be too expensive to conduct. In these settings, the study of stroke prevalence using door-to-door surveys and the STEPwise approach to stroke surveillance (WHO STEPS-stroke) for studying stroke incidence facilitated by verbal autopsy data collection may be used as alternative sources of information [5]. Using all available observational data from various sources, the GBD studies provide a comprehensive picture of the current global burden of stroke, as well as temporal trends in age-standardized stroke incidence, prevalence, DALYs and mortality in 1990, 2005, 2010 and 2013 [6].

Worldwide Burden of Stroke

The first global estimates produced by the GBD 2010 showed that an estimated 16.9 million strokes occurred in 2010, with 69% of these occurring in low- and middle-income countries [7]. The study also showed that in 2010, stroke was the second-most common cause of death and the third-most common cause of DALYs in the world. Between 1990 and 2010, the global incidence of stroke increased slightly, but not significantly, while the prevalence of stroke increased significantly by 16%. Both DALYs and mortality rates declined significantly over this period. However, in terms of absolute numbers, incident stroke, prevalent stroke, DALYs and deaths increased globally by 68%, 84%, 12% and 26%, respectively, with the greatest increases seen in those aged 85 or older. In terms of the stroke subtypes, estimates from the GBD 2010 showed that globally in absolute numbers there were 11.6 million incident ischaemic and 5.3 million incident haemorrhagic strokes, with 2.8 million deaths from ischaemic stroke and 3 million deaths from haemorrhagic stroke [8]. There was a significant increase in the incidence rate of haemorrhagic stroke since 1990.

Trends in stroke burden differed between high-income and low- and middle-income countries. In high-income countries, stroke incidence declined significantly by 12%. In low- and middle-income countries, there was a significant increase in stroke incidence in the younger age group of 20–64 years of 18%. There was a significant increase in stroke prevalence in high-income countries of 27%. DALY rates were reduced in high-income countries by 36%, and low- and middle-income countries by 22%. Similarly, death rates declined significantly in both high-income countries by 37%, and in low-and middle-income countries by 20%.

GBD 2013 Findings

The GBD estimates of stroke burden were updated in the GBD 2013 study. These findings showed that stroke resulted in close to 6.5 million deaths in 2013, almost 2.5 million more than in 1990 [9]. Age-adjusted DALYs, incidence, prevalence and mortality are reported separately for ischaemic stroke and haemorrhagic stroke (Fig. **3.1**) [6, 10]. Between 1990 and 2013, significant decreases were found in the global incidence, DALY and mortality rates of ischaemic stroke, while for haemorrhagic stroke, incidence and prevalence rates increased (mortality statistically non-significant) and DALY and mortality rates declined. Global estimates of age-standardized DALYs and mortality for total stroke, ischaemic stroke and haemorrhagic stroke for 2013 are shown in Figs. (**3.2a-f**). In terms of absolute numbers, there were 6.9 million cases of ischaemic stroke and 3.2 million cases of haemorrhagic stroke, a significant increase from 1990.

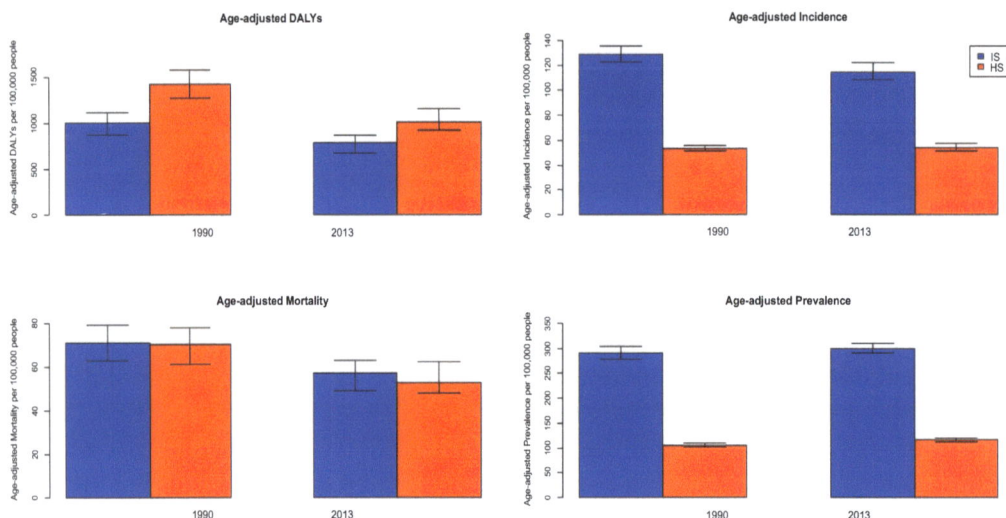

Fig. (3.1). Global trends in ischaemic stroke (IS) and haemorrhagic stroke (HS) burden between 1990 and 2013.
Source: Global Burden of Disease Study 2013 *(1)*http://vizhub.healthdata.org/gbd-compare/).

2. ARE THERE DIFFERENCES IN LOW- AND MIDDLE-INCOME COUNTRIES COMPARED TO HIGH-INCOME COUNTRIES?

Ischaemic and haemorrhagic stroke death rate and stroke burden (DALY) rate were 2.0-fold higher in low- and middle-income countries, an increase from the 1.4 and 1.6-fold difference for death rate and stroke burden rate, respectively, in 1990. (Figs. **3.3a-f**) show death and disease burden rates per 100 000 for global, low- and middle-income and high-income countries by age. Death and stroke burden rates are significantly higher, particularly in those over age 75 in low- and middle-income countries for haemorrhagic stroke. Stroke burden rates for all strokes, but particularly for haemorrhagic stroke, are significantly higher in low- and middle-income countries in those aged 50 or older. Compared to high-income countries, the ischaemic stroke death and stroke burden rates were 1.5-fold higher in low- and middle-income countries, while for haemorrhagic stroke, stroke death and stroke burden rates were 3.2-fold higher.

Cerebrovascular disease
Both sexes, Age-standardized, 2013, DALYs per 100,000

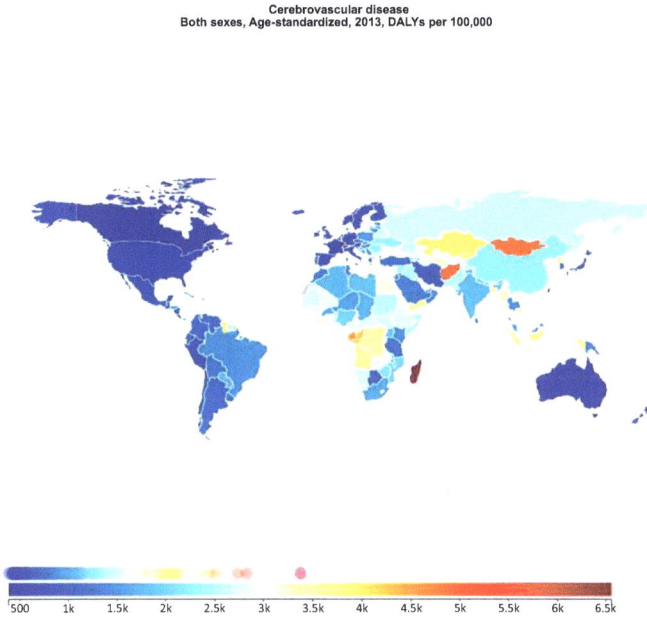

Fig. (3.2a).

Cerebrovascular disease
Both sexes, Age-standardized, 2013, Deaths per 100,000

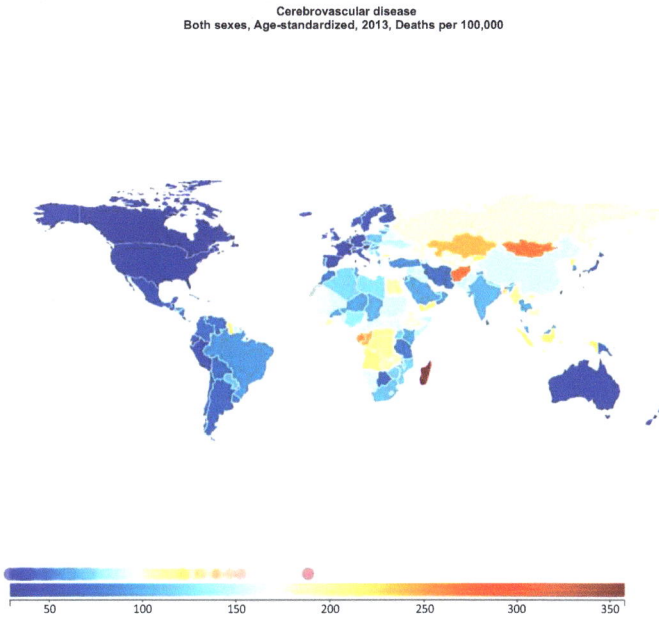

Fig. (3.2b).

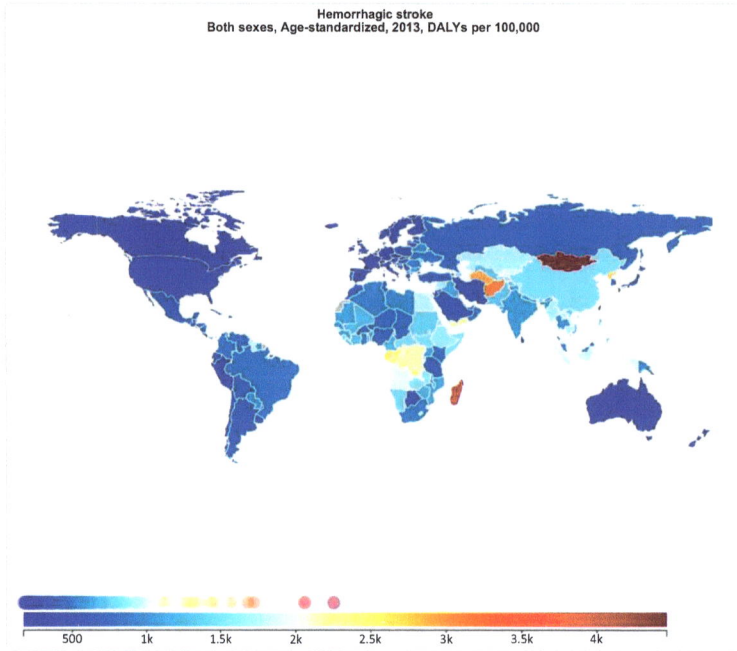

Fig. (3.2c).

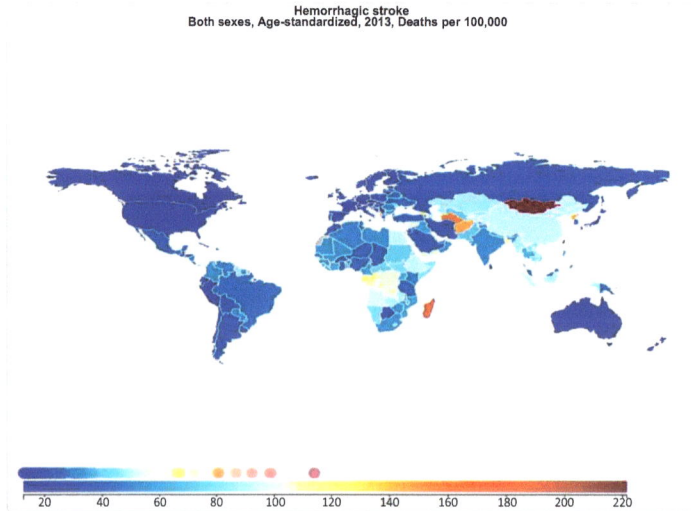

Fig. (3.2d).

Ischemic stroke
Both sexes, Age-standardized, 2013, DALYs per 100,000

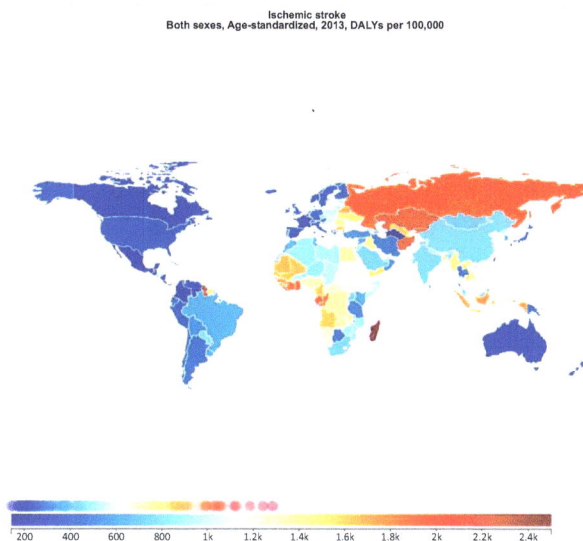

Fig. (3.2e).

Ischemic stroke
Both sexes, Age-standardized, 2013, Deaths per 100,000

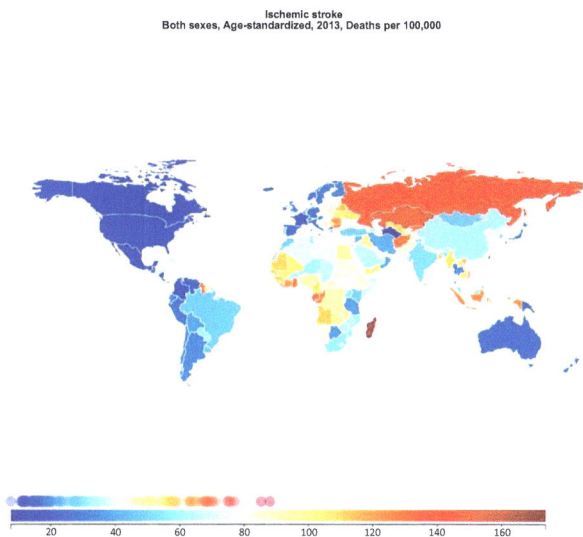

Fig. (3.2f).

Figs. (3.2a-f). Age-standardized mortality for stroke in 2013.
Source: Global Burden of Disease Study 2013 *(1)*. http://vizhub.healthdata.org/gbd-compare/).

The prevalence rate of ischaemic stroke was significantly higher in high-income countries by 3.7-fold, while the prevalence of haemorrhagic stroke was similar in low- and middle-income countries and high-income countries. Between 1990 and 2013, death from ischaemic stroke and haemorrhagic stroke declined significantly in high-income countries, but not in low- and middle-income countries. Notably, the prevalence of both ischaemic stroke and haemorrhagic stroke increased significantly between 1990 and 2013 in high-income countries, but not in low- and middle-income countries.

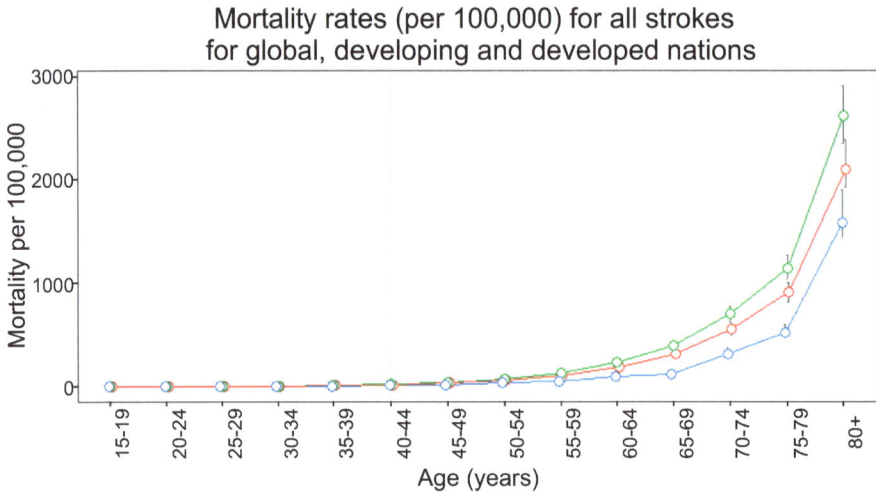

Fig. (3.3a).

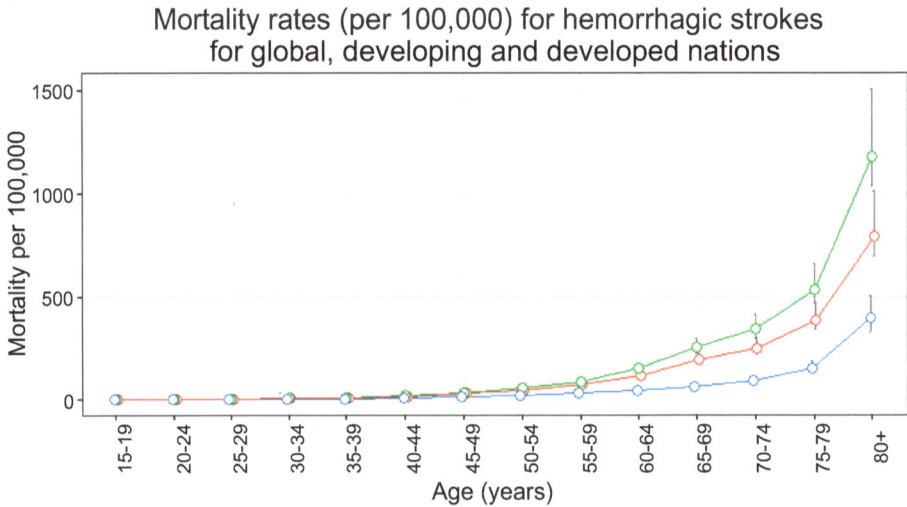

Fig. (3.3b).

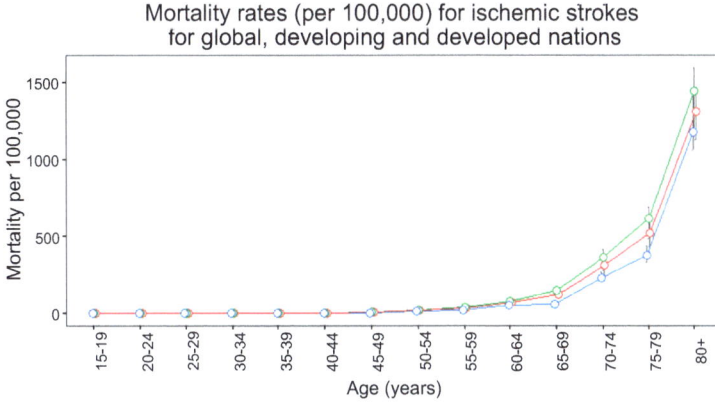

Fig. (3.3c).

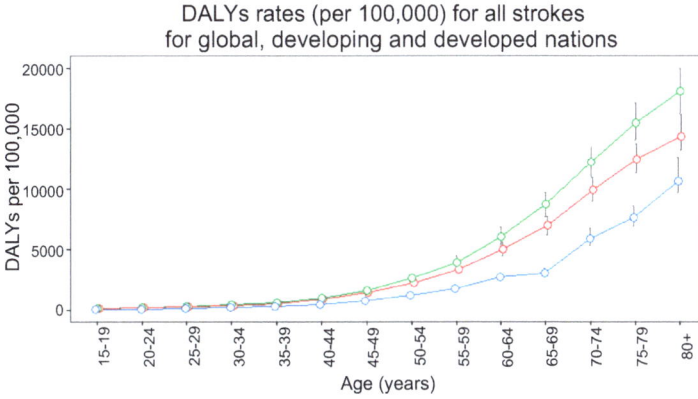

Fig. (3.3d).

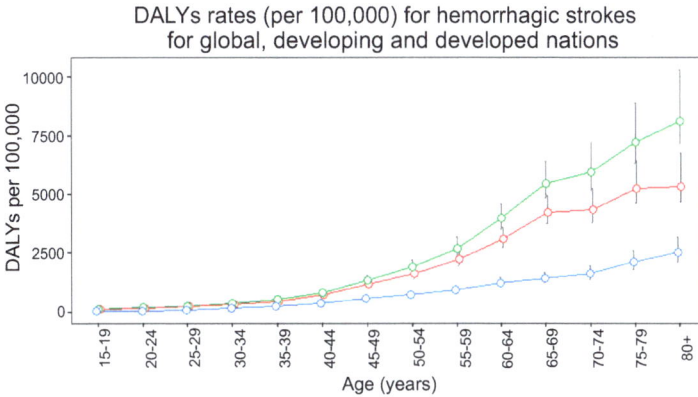

Fig. (3.3e).

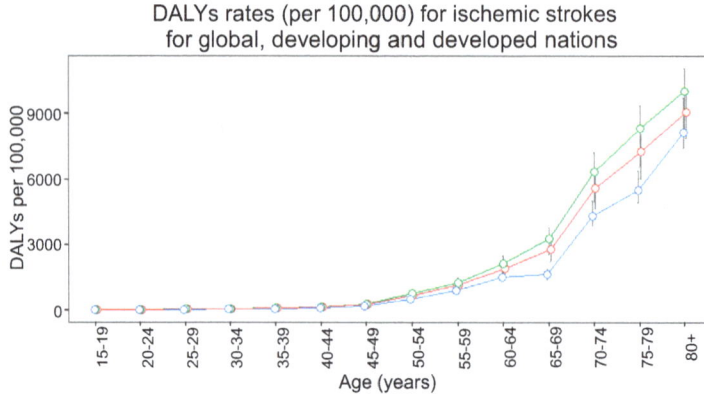

DALYs rates (per 100,000) for ischemic strokes
for global, developing and developed nations

Fig. (3.3f).

Figs. (3.3a-f). Mortality rates for strokes.
Notes:
Red line = global
Green line = developing countries
Blue line = developed countries
Source: Seattle, United States: Institute for Health Metrics and Evaluation (IHME); 2016.

Stroke in Younger Adults

In younger adults aged 20–64, the prevalence of ischaemic stroke was almost 7.3 million and the prevalence of haemorrhagic stroke was just over 3.7 million, representing almost 40% of ischaemic stroke and just over 50% of the total prevalent haemorrhagic strokes. Compared to low- and middle-income countries, the prevalence rate of both ischaemic stroke and haemorrhagic stroke in this age group was significantly higher in high-income countries. From 1990 to 2013, there were significant increases in prevalence rates of both ischaemic stroke and haemorrhagic stroke in all countries. In 20–64 year olds, there were almost 1.5 million deaths due to stroke in 2013, with a significantly higher number of deaths due to haemorrhagic stroke than deaths due to ischaemic stroke. The death rate as well as the number of deaths were significantly higher in low- and middle-income countries than in high-income countries.

Between 1990 and 2013, globally there was a 26% increase in prevalent strokes (22% ischaemic stroke and 36% haemorrhagic stroke). In contrast, the death rates for all strokes declined in high-income countries. Stroke burden, as measured by DALYs, increased by 24% globally in the 20–64 year age group (20% for ischaemic stroke and 37.3% for haemorrhagic stroke). However, stroke burden rates declined significantly in high-income countries, with a similar trend (non-significant) seen in low- and middle-income countries.

3. ARE THERE SEX DIFFERENCES IN STROKE BURDEN?

The GBD 2013 studies produced estimates for stroke incidence, prevalence, death and stroke burden separately for males and females. In 2013 in females, the incidence rate of ischaemic stroke was 98.8 (92.1–106.6) per 100 000 and 45.4 (42.3–104.26) for haemorrhagic stroke. The incidence rate of both ischaemic stroke at 132.7 (125.3–142.7) and haemorrhagic stroke at 64.9 (59.868.5) per 100 000 in males was significantly higher than in females.

Similarly, prevalence rates in 2013 for both ischaemic stroke and haemorrhagic stroke were significantly higher in males. Prevalence rates of ischaemic stroke were significantly higher by 3.8-fold and 3.6-fold in high-income countries compared to low- and middle-income countries for females and males, respectively. Prevalence rates for haemorrhagic stroke were 1.5-fold and 1.1-fold higher for males in high-income countries and low- and middle-income countries, respectively.

Stroke burden rates in males were significantly higher for haemorrhagic stroke compared to females. While death rates were not significantly different for ischaemic stroke in males and females, females had a significantly higher death rate for haemorrhagic stroke compared to males. Compared to 1990, incidence rates overall were lower in 2013 for both males and females, but this change was only significant for ischaemic stroke in females. Death rates of both ischaemic and haemorrhagic strokes reduced for both males and females.

4. WHY SHOULD STROKE PREVENTION BE A PRIORITY?

The GBD 2013 updates confirm that stroke continues to have a major and increasing impact on global health, particularly in developing regions of the world. While mortality rates have declined, prevalent rates are increasing, meaning that millions of people are left with some degree of disability. Stroke, along with ischaemic heart disease, are important contributors of death in middle age (50–75 years), and stroke is in the top three causes of years of life lost in high-income countries [1]. The majority of strokes are preventable [11, 12]. Therefore, the impact can be significantly reduced with primary prevention. For these reasons, stroke prevention should be a public health priority worldwide.

Moreover, as the majority of strokes do not result in death although they leave most survivors with some level of disability, the impact of stroke on disability must be equally considered. Stroke ranks number three among the most common causes of disease burden after ischaemic heart disease and lung and respiratory infections [13]. Many survivors become dependent on others for most or all of their activities of daily living, which has huge physical, psychological and economic implications. Stroke also increases the risk of conditions such as dementia and depression, compounding its already devastating effects [14].

The impact of stroke extends to the affected person's family as the majority of stroke survivors, many with physical impairments as well as cognitive and speech impairment, return home and are often cared for by their spouse or other family members. Caring for stroke survivors, particularly for those with severe impairment, causes significant carer burden [15]. The increasing numbers of stroke survivors and people affected by stroke throughout the world are greatly overstretching the already limited health-care resources. The most pertinent solution to the problem is effective primary stroke prevention.

5. WHAT ARE THE CURRENT STROKE PREVENTION STRATEGIES?

Population-wide Strategies

The currently recommended primary stroke prevention strategies include population-wide and high-risk prevention strategies. The World Health Assembly has endorsed a global monitoring framework and a set of targets for NCDs, including stroke [17]. The overarching target is to reduce the risk of premature NCD deaths (between ages 30 and 70) by 25% by 2025, by targeting six key risk factors and two health systems-related targets (25 by 25 target) [16, 17]. These targets are all relevant to stroke risk – raised blood pressure, diabetes mellitus, obesity, tobacco use, harmful use of alcohol, sodium intake and physical inactivity. An additional target of medical management of high cardiovascular disease risk individuals is also included. Of the behavioural risk factors of relevance to stroke, the targets include: (i) a minimum 10% relative reduction in harmful use of alcohol and prevalence of inadequate physical activity; (ii) a 30% relative reduction in the average intake of sodium; (iii) a 30% relative reduction in the prevalence of tobacco use in adults; (iv) a 25% relative reduction in the prevalence of raised blood pressure; and (v) halting the rise in diabetes and obesity [16]. In addition, national response targets include providing drug therapy and counselling to at least 50% of eligible people and 80% affordability of basic technologies and essential medicines in public and private facilities.

In population-wide prevention strategies, interventions used to reduce exposure to risk factors are applied to the whole population irrespective of their baseline risk or health conditions. This is the most cost-effective prevention strategy because it targets not only stroke, but also other major NCDs that share common risk factors with stroke such as myocardial infarction, dementia, diabetes mellitus and cancer [14]. Even a minor shift in the distribution of risk factors in the population can result in reductions in the incidence of these disorders [18, 19]. A systematic review and meta-analysis of randomized trials of modest salt reduction has shown that there is a significant association in reduced salt intake and a fall in systolic blood pressure. Such a fall in blood pressure would reduce the risk of stroke [20]. Other examples of this strategy include smoking cessation campaigns (plain packaging, warning messages, *etc.*) [21] and legislative changes (*e.g.* tobacco taxes, banning smoking in public places) [22] that have been shown to be very successful in many countries. Despite increased efforts towards population-wide primary prevention over the past few decades, gaps in prevention persist.

High-risk Strategy

In the high-risk prevention strategy, people are categorized as being at low, moderate or high absolute risk of stroke and other cardiovascular diseases. Interventions such as prescription of medications are aimed primarily at people with moderate to high risk of cardiovascular disease. This approach is very cost effective compared to targeting of single risk factors and has been shown to be affordable for all low- and middle-income countries. It has been implemented in many low- and middle-income countries through integrated primary health care programmes, using the WHO Package of Essential NCD Interventions (WHO PEN) [23]. The global NCD target 8 (see Table **2.5**), to reduce heart attacks and strokes aims to improve the coverage of drug treatment and counselling to prevent heart attacks and strokes in people with raised cardiovascular risk and established disease.

Several issues need to be given due consideration for successful implementation of the high-risk strategy. First, labelling people as being at low or moderate cardiovascular disease risk may give them a false sense of reassurance of their safety from cardiovascular disease. To avoid this and to motivate people to make behavioural changes, high-risk strategies should always be complemented with population-wide prevention and health promotion strategies. Some people may have mild hypertension, but still have a low absolute risk of cardiovascular disease. They require counselling for behavioural change and medications if blood pressure fails to respond to reduction of harmful use of alcohol, healthy diet (low in salt and rich in fruit and vegetables) and regular physical activity [24]. Second, evaluating absolute cardiovascular disease risk may require lab tests (*e.g.* blood lipid and blood glucose tests) and visiting a medical professional, thus imposing a cost to people. In resource-poor settings, risk stratification tools that use non-la--based indicators may need to be used. Finally, screening the population for cardiovascular disease risk by itself has not been shown to reduce incidence or mortality from cardiovascular disease [25, 26]. Screening always needs to be complemented with population-wide strategies to reduce exposure of the whole population to behavioural risk factors and health system reforms to strengthen primary care.

6. WHAT ARE THE GAPS IN STROKE PREVENTION STRATEGIES AND HOW CAN THEY BE ADDRESSED?

There are huge gaps in population-wide stroke prevention strategies across all countries in the world, and particularly between high-income countries and low- and middle-income countries. Although, there is still no country in the world where population-wide stroke prevention strategies are implemented in full, in selected regions of some high-income countries (*e.g.* North Karelia, Japan, United States) such strategies are being implemented and smoking cessation campaigns are being implemented in the majority of high-income countries. In contrast, in low- and middle-income countries, implementation of population-wide strategies to address stroke (and other NCDs) is weak. These countries are experiencing a significant increase in exposure to smoking and other behavioural risks for stroke (*e.g.* unhealthy diet, harmful use of alcohol and physical inactivity). The ever-increasing global burden of stroke, especially in low- and middle-income countries, necessitates an urgent implementation of very cost-effective population-wide strategies (see Table **2.3**) to reduce population exposure to behavioural risk factors.

The other approach to primary stroke prevention is a high-risk approach when people are screened for their cardiovascular disease risk and those identified with high risk are offered treatment to reduce their total cardiovascular risk [23]. This includes not only treating hypertension, but also addressing diabetes, raised blood lipids, tobacco use, harmful use of alcohol, unhealthy diet and physical inactivity. Weak health systems at the primary health care level are a major barrier for implementing the high-risk strategy in low- and middle-income countries [27]. Vertical programmes to manage hypertension are neither cost effective nor sustainable for resource-constrained settings. What is required is to give priority to very cost-effective high-impact total cardiovascular risk reduction ("best buy", see Table **2.3**), in moving towards universal health coverage and to address health-system and coverage gaps through mechanisms that are sensitive to specific country contexts [27, 28].

The challenges associated with implementing the high-risk strategy has prompted researchers to find better solutions to improve the effectiveness of this strategy. One such example is the use of mobile technologies (apps) for managing risk factors (*e.g.* smoking cessation *via* text messaging and weight reduction) that have been tested for their effectiveness in randomized clinical trials [29]. However, there is a need for larger trials and the evaluation of the long-term impact of these interventions.

Another example of such an approach specifically designed for primary stroke prevention using mobile technology is the Stroke Riskometer app. This app uses demographic and health information entered into the app by the user to calculate not only an absolute risk, but also the relative risk of stroke for people aged 20 or older. The app contributes to motivating people with low to moderate absolute risk to control their risk factors, and educates people about stroke, its warning signs and ways to reduce their risk factors. By empowering people to control their risk and providing means for such control on an individual level, the Stroke Riskometer app is recognized as a new paradigm in stroke prevention [30, 31]. The app has been fully validated and is currently being tested in a randomized controlled trial in New Zealand. Another promising option that has the potential to improve stroke prevention is the use of a polypill – for example, a pill consisting of a combination of several medications (blood pressure lowering medications, aspirin and statins). If shown to improve outcomes and to be safe and very cost effective in ongoing trials, the polypill can also contribute to stroke prevention, including through improvement of patient compliance and ease of administration.

7. WHAT ARE THE CURRENT SURGICAL STROKE PREVENTION STRATEGIES?

Revascularization (improving blood flow) of the extracranial (outside the skull bone) and intracranial (inside the skull bone) carotid and vertebral arteries

About one fifth of ischaemic strokes are caused by atherothromboembolism of the origin of the ipsilateral (same side) extracranial internal carotid artery (a large artery that traverses the neck to supply blood to the brain). Treating extracranial internal carotid artery atherosclerosis by means of revascularization therapy such as carotid endarterectomy (surgical removal of part of the inner lining of an artery, together with any obstructive deposits) or carotid artery stenting (placing a small mesh tube to improve blood flow), and medical therapy such as cardiovascular risk factor control and antiplatelet therapy reduces the risk of further stroke [32 - 34].

The benefits of carotid revascularization therapy are greater in patients with carotid artery atherosclerosis that is recently symptomatic (*i.e.* caused recent carotid-territory brain or retinal ischaemia) than neurologically asymptomatic. This is because the risk of further stroke is considerably greater after recently symptomatic (*i.e.* active or unstable) carotid atherosclerosis than with asymptomatic (*i.e.* inactive or stable) carotid atherosclerosis, despite higher risks of perioperative stroke or death with symptomatic (3–7%) than asymptomatic

(1–2%) carotid atherosclerosis. Indeed, recent improvements in medical therapies, particularly antiplatelet therapy and blood pressure control, have resulted in a very low average annual risk of any ipsilateral ischaemic stroke distal to ≥50% asymptomatic carotid stenosis (as low as 0.34%), thus obviating the need for additional carotid revascularization therapy in many neurologically asymptomatic patients (patients who did not have a transient ischaemic attack or stroke) [35, 36].

Symptomatic Extracranial Carotid Artery Stenosis (Narrowing)

Carotid Endarterectomy plus Optimal Medical Therapy versus Optimal Medical Therapy Alone

Carotid endarterectomy in patients with recent symptomatic extracranial atherosclerotic carotid stenosis reduced the risk of stroke or death at five years (by half in patients with 70–99% stenosis, and a quarter with 50–69% stenosis), when added to medical therapy in trials conducted 25 years ago) [33]. The benefits of carotid endarterectomy plus optimal medical therapy were greatest in surgically-fit patients with a high 5-year risk of ipsilateral stroke (>20%). Increased degree of narrowing, advanced age, male sex and recent transient ischaemic attack or stroke were associated with increasing benefit from surgery. These results are generalizable only to surgically-fit patients operated on by surgeons with low complication rates (less than 7% risk of stroke and death). In contrast, patients with a lower risk of stroke did not benefit significantly from carotid endarterectomy because the benefit of surgery in the longer-term prevention of stroke did not justify the perioperative risk of stroke or death.

Carotid Artery Stenting versus Carotid Endarterectomy

Carotid artery stenting for symptomatic carotid stenosis increases the risk of peri-procedural stroke or death compared with endarterectomy [34]. This is mainly because the risk of peri-procedural stroke or death associated with carotid artery stenting increases with increasing age of patients, particularly over age 70, whereas the periprocedural risk of stroke and death in patients undergoing endarterectomy does not increase with increasing age [34, 37]. However, carotid artery stenting is associated with lower risks of peri-operative myocardial infarction (heart attacks), cranial nerve palsy (paralysis of nerves) and access site haematomas compared to endarterectomy [34]. The long-term rates of fatal or disabling stroke, composite of major vascular events, and functional outcome are similar after stenting and endarterectomy [38, 39].

Timing of Carotid Revascularization after Symptomatic Carotid Stenosis

Carotid revascularization should be performed early, within the first week after stroke or a transient ischaemic attack of the brain, when the risk of recurrent stroke is highest. The risk of perioperative stroke is about 3.3% after early endarterectomy, and about 4.8% after early stenting. The risks may be higher with hyperacute surgery performed within 48 hours after symptom onset [40].

8. WHAT ARE THE FUTURE DIRECTIONS IN SURGICAL PREVENTION OF STROKE?

Given the advances in medical therapies over the past 25 years and concurrent lower rates of recurrent stroke in patients with symptomatic carotid stenosis treated medically, the second European Carotid Surgery Trial (ECST-2) is currently comparing the risks and benefits of adding immediate carotid surgery (or stenting) to modern medical therapy in patients with symptomatic or asymptomatic atherosclerotic carotid artery stenosis at low and intermediate risk for stroke. It is hypothesized that in patients with carotid stenosis at low and intermediate risk for stroke, optimal medical therapy alone is as effective in the long-term prevention of cerebral infarction and myocardial infarction as revascularization and optimal medical therapy combined.

Symptomatic Intracranial Carotid and Vertebrobasilar Stenosis, and Extracranial Vertebral Stenosis

Stenting of recently symptomatic atherosclerotic intracranial stenosis and extracranial vertebral stenosis is associated with unacceptable peri-procedural risks of stroke or death that preclude its use compared to intensive medical therapy [41 - 43].

There is also no benefit of flow-augmentation extracranial to intracranial bypass surgery over medical therapy for patients with intracranial artery occlusion and severe hemodynamic impairment because of the increased perioperative morbidity [44].

Asymptomatic Carotid Stenosis

Carotid Endarterectomy plus Optimal Medical Therapy versus Optimal Medical Therapy Alone

Two trials that recruited a total of 1036 patients with asymptomatic carotid stenosis before 2000 showed that carotid endarterectomy was associated with increased risk of perioperative stroke, compared to medical therapy alone [45, 46].

However, in the longer term, three trials that recruited a total of 5223 patients before 2000 showed the carotid endarterectomy was associated with a lower risk of stroke than with medical therapy alone, but with no significant difference in any stroke or death. Given recent advances in optimal medical therapy since patients were recruited in the above trials (in the 1980s and 1990s), it is uncertain whether any carotid revascularization procedure confers additional benefit in preventing ipsilateral carotid territory ischaemic stroke in asymptomatic patients with significant carotid stenosis.

Carotid Artery Stenting versus Carotid Endarterectomy

Three trials have compared carotid artery stenting plus medical therapy *versus* carotid endarterectomy plus medical therapy [39, 47, 48]. After deducting the perioperative risks of stroke or death within 30 days of carotid artery stenting (about 3%) or endarterectomy (about 2%), the long-term risks of stroke or death are similar with stenting and endarterectomy for asymptomatic carotid stenosis. Evidence is insufficient to clearly support one interventional strategy over another in adults with asymptomatic carotid stenosis.

Screening for Asymptomatic Carotid Stenosis

Given the low prevalence of severe carotid stenosis in the general population, screening asymptomatic people may result in more strokes than it prevents [49].

CONCLUDING REMARKS

Despite the fact that stroke risk factors are well known and several prevention strategies are in place, the increasing burden of stroke implies that stroke prevention strategies have not been effectively implemented worldwide. Strokes cause long-term disability and death. The chances of dying are much higher with subsequent strokes, which often occur within one year of the first attack. A public health approach for prevention and control of stroke needs to combine a population-wide strategy for reduction of exposure to behavioural risk factors with a health systems strengthening strategy for individual risk reduction of high-risk individuals using a total risk approach.

CONFLICT OF INTEREST

The authors declare no conflict of interest, financial or otherwise.

ACKNOWLEDGEMENTS

Ms AvisAnne Julien is thanked for copy-editing.

REFERENCES

[1]   Naghavi M, Wang H, Lozano R, *et al.* GBD 2013 Mortality and Causes of Death Collaborators. Global, regional, and national age-sex specific all-cause and cause-specific mortality for 240 causes of death, 1990-2013: a systematic analysis for the Global Burden of Disease Study 2013. Lancet 2015; 385(9963): 117-71.
[http://dx.doi.org/10.1016/S0140-6736(14)61682-2] [PMID: 25530442]

[2]   Strong K, Mathers C, Bonita R. Preventing stroke: saving lives around the world. Lancet Neurology 2007; 6: 182-7.
[http://dx.doi.org/10.1016/S1474-4422(07)70031-5]

[3]   Feigin V, Norrving B, Krishnamurthi R, Barker-Collo S, Wang W, Fu H, Eds. Stroke Riskometer app: a new promising approach for primary stroke prevention and epidemiological research on stroke and other major non-communicable disorders (NCDs) across the globe. Int J Stroke 2015; 10: 101-2.

[4]   Sudlow CLM, Warlow CP. Comparing stroke incidence worldwide: What makes studies comparable? Stroke 1996; 27(3): 550-8.

[5]   Feigin VL. Stroke in developing countries: Can the epidemic be stopped and outcomes improved? Lancet Neurology 2007; 6(2): 94-7.

[6]   Roth GA, Johnson CO, Nguyen G, *et al.* Methods for estimating the global burden of cerebrovascular diseases. Neuroepidemiology 2015; 45(3): 146-51.
[http://dx.doi.org/10.1159/000441083] [PMID: 26505980]

[7]   Lozano R, Naghavi M, Foreman K, *et al.* Global and regional mortality from 235 causes of death for 20 age groups in 1990 and 2010: a systematic analysis for the Global Burden of Disease Study 2010. Lancet 2012; 380(9859): 2095-128.
[http://dx.doi.org/10.1016/S0140-6736(12)61728-0] [PMID: 23245604]

[8]   Krishnamurthi RV, Feigin VL, Forouzanfar MH, *et al.* Global and regional burden of first-ever ischaemic and haemorrhagic stroke during 1990-2010: findings from the Global Burden of Disease Study 2010. Lancet Glob Health 2013; 1(5): e259-81.
[http://dx.doi.org/10.1016/S2214-109X(13)70089-5] [PMID: 25104492]

[9]   Feigin VL, Krishnamurthi RV, Parmar P, *et al.* Update on the global burden of ischemic and hemorrhagic stroke in 1990–2013: the GBD 2013 study. Neuroepidemiology 2015; 45(3): 161-76.
[http://dx.doi.org/10.1159/000441085] [PMID: 26505981]

[10]   Mensah GA, Sacco RL, Vickrey BG, *et al.* From data to action: neuroepidemiology informs implementation research for global stroke prevention and treatment. Neuroepidemiology 2015; 45(3): 221-9.
[http://dx.doi.org/10.1159/000441105] [PMID: 26505615]

[11]   Feigin VL, Krishnamurthi R. Stroke is largely preventable across the globe: where to next? Lancet 2016; 388(10046): 733-4.
[http://dx.doi.org/10.1016/S0140-6736(16)30679-1] [PMID: 27431357]

[12]   O'Donnell MJ, Xavier D, Liu L, *et al.* Risk factors for ischaemic and intracerebral haemorrhagic stroke in 22 countries (the INTERSTROKE study): a case-control study. Lancet 2010; 376(9735): 112-23.
[http://dx.doi.org/10.1016/S0140-6736(10)60834-3] [PMID: 20561675]

[13]   Murray CJ, Vos T, Lozano R, *et al.* Disability-adjusted life years (DALYs) for 291 diseases and injuries in 21 regions, 1990-2010: a systematic analysis for the Global Burden of Disease Study 2010. Lancet 2012; 380(9859): 2197-223.
[http://dx.doi.org/10.1016/S0140-6736(12)61689-4] [PMID: 23245608]

[14]   Gorelick PB, Farooq MU, Min J. Population-based approaches for reducing stroke risk. Expert Rev Cardiovasc Ther 2015; 13(1): 49-56.
[http://dx.doi.org/10.1586/14779072.2015.987128] [PMID: 25434376]

[15]   Quinn K, Murray C, Malone C. Spousal experiences of coping with and adapting to caregiving for a partner who has a stroke: a meta-synthesis of qualitative research. Disabil Rehabil 2014; 36(3): 185-98.
[http://dx.doi.org/10.3109/09638288.2013.783630] [PMID: 23597001]

[16]   Draft comprehensive global monitoring framework and targets for the prevention and control of noncommunicable diseases. Geneva: World Health Organization 2013.

[17]   Sacco RL, Roth GA, Reddy KS, *et al.* The heart of 25 by 25: Achieving the goal of reducing global and regional premature deaths from cardiovascular diseases and stroke: A modeling study from the American Heart Association and World Heart Federation. Circulation 2016; 133(23): e674-90.
[http://dx.doi.org/10.1161/CIR.0000000000000395] [PMID: 27162236]

[18]   Younus A, Aneni EC, Spatz ES, *et al.* A systematic review of the prevalence and outcomes of ideal cardiovascular health in US and non-US populations. Mayo Clin Proc 2016; 91(5): 649-70.
[http://dx.doi.org/10.1016/j.mayocp.2016.01.019] [PMID: 27040086]

[19]   Asaria P, Chisholm D, Mathers C, Ezzati M, Beaglehole R. Chronic disease prevention: health effects and financial costs of strategies to reduce salt intake and control tobacco use. Lancet 2007; 370(9604): 2044-53.
[http://dx.doi.org/10.1016/S0140-6736(07)61698-5] [PMID: 18063027]

[20]   He FJ, Li J, MacGregor GA. Effect of longer term modest salt reduction on blood pressure: Cochrane systematic review and meta-analysis of randomised trials. BMJ (Online) 2013; 346(7903)

[21]   Mons U, Müezzinler A, Gellert C, Schöttker B, Abnet CC, Bobak M, *et al.* Impact of smoking and smoking cessation on cardiovascular events and mortality among older adults: meta-analysis of individual participant data from prospective cohort studies of the CHANCES consortium BMJ (Online) 2015; 350
[http://dx.doi.org/10.1136/bmj.h1551]

[22]   Asma S, Warren W, Althomsons S, Wisotzky M, Woollery T, Henson R. Addressing the chronic disease burden with tobacco control programs. Public Health Rep 2004; 119(3): 253-62.
[http://dx.doi.org/10.1016/j.phr.2004.04.004] [PMID: 15158104]

[23]   Implementation tools: package of essential noncommunicable (WHO PEN) disease interventions for primary health care in low-resource settings. 2013. Available at: http://www.who.int/cardiovascular_diseases/publications/implementation_tools_WHO_PEN/en/

[24]   Dalton AR, Soljak M, Samarasundera E, Millett C, Majeed A. Prevalence of cardiovascular disease risk amongst the population eligible for the NHS Health Check Programme. Eur J Prev Cardiol 2013; 20(1): 142-50.
[http://dx.doi.org/10.1177/1741826711428797] [PMID: 22058079]

[25]   Krogsbøll LT, Jørgensen KJ, Grønhøj Larsen C, Gøtzsche PC. General health checks in adults for reducing morbidity and mortality from disease: Cochrane systematic review and meta-analysis. BMJ (Online) 2012; 345(7884)

[26]   Jørgensen T, Jacobsen RK, Toft U, Aadahl M, Glümer C, Pisinger C. Effect of screening and lifestyle counselling on incidence of ischaemic heart disease in general population: Inter99 randomised trial. BMJ (Online) 2014; 348

[27]   Global status report on noncommunicable diseases 2014. Geneva: World Health Organization 2014.

[28]   Mendis S, O'Brien E, Seedat YK, Yusuf S. Hypertension and diabetes: entry points for prevention and control of the global cardiovascular epidemic. Int J Hypertens 2013; 2013: 878460.
[http://dx.doi.org/10.1155/2013/878460]

[29]   Brendryen H, Kraft P. Happy ending: a randomized controlled trial of a digital multi-media smoking cessation intervention. Addiction 2008; 103(3): 478-84.
[http://dx.doi.org/10.1111/j.1360-0443.2007.02119.x] [PMID: 18269367]

[30]   Parmar P, Krishnamurthi R, Ikram MA, *et al.* The Stroke Riskometer(TM) App: validation of a data collection tool and stroke risk predictor. Int J Stroke 2015; 10(2): 231-44.
[http://dx.doi.org/10.1111/ijs.12411] [PMID: 25491651]

[31]   Feigin VL, Krishnamurthi R, Bhattacharjee R, *et al.* New strategy to reduce the global burden of stroke. Stroke 2015; 46(6): 1740-7.
[http://dx.doi.org/10.1161/STROKEAHA.115.008222] [PMID: 25882050]

[32]   Raman G, Moorthy D, Hadar N, *et al.* Management strategies for asymptomatic carotid stenosis: a systematic review and meta-analysis. Ann Intern Med 2013; 158(9): 676-85.
[http://dx.doi.org/10.7326/0003-4819-158-9-201305070-00007] [PMID: 23648949]

[33]   Rerkasem K, Rothwell PM. Carotid endarterectomy for symptomatic carotid stenosis. Cochrane Database Syst Rev 2011; (4): CD001081.
[PMID: 21491381]

[34]   Bonati LH, Lyrer P, Ederle J, Featherstone R, Brown MM. Percutaneous transluminal balloon angioplasty and stenting for carotid artery stenosis. Cochrane Database Syst Rev 2012; (9): CD000515.
[PMID: 22972047]

[35]   Marquardt L, Geraghty OC, Mehta Z, Rothwell PM. Low risk of ipsilateral stroke in patients with asymptomatic carotid stenosis on best medical treatment: a prospective, population-based study. Stroke 2010; 41(1): e11-7.
[http://dx.doi.org/10.1161/STROKEAHA.109.561837] [PMID: 19926843]

[36]   King A, Shipley M, Markus H. The effect of medical treatments on stroke risk in asymptomatic carotid stenosis. Stroke 2013; 44(2): 542-6.
[http://dx.doi.org/10.1161/STROKEAHA.112.673608] [PMID: 23192761]

[37]   Howard G, Roubin GS, Jansen O, *et al.* Association between age and risk of stroke or death from carotid endarterectomy and carotid stenting: a meta-analysis of pooled patient data from four randomised trials. Lancet 2016; 387(10025): 1305-11.
[http://dx.doi.org/10.1016/S0140-6736(15)01309-4] [PMID: 26880122]

[38]   Bonati LH, Dobson J, Featherstone RL, *et al.* Long-term outcomes after stenting *versus* endarterectomy for treatment of symptomatic carotid stenosis: the International Carotid Stenting Study (ICSS) randomised trial. Lancet 2015; 385(9967): 529-38.
[http://dx.doi.org/10.1016/S0140-6736(14)61184-3] [PMID: 25453443]

[39]   Brott TG, Howard G, Roubin GS, *et al.* Long-term results of stenting *versus* endarterectomy for carotid-artery stenosis. N Engl J Med 2016; 374(11): 1021-31.
[http://dx.doi.org/10.1056/NEJMoa1505215] [PMID: 26890472]

[40]   De Rango P, Brown MM, Chaturvedi S, *et al.* Summary of evidence on early carotid intervention for recently symptomatic stenosis based on meta-analysis of current risks. Stroke 2015; 46(12): 3423-36.
[http://dx.doi.org/10.1161/STROKEAHA.115.010764] [PMID: 26470773]

[41]   Compter A, van der Worp HB, Schonewille WJ, *et al.* Stenting *versus* medical treatment in patients with symptomatic vertebral artery stenosis: a randomised open-label phase 2 trial. Lancet Neurol 2015; 14(6): 606-14.
[http://dx.doi.org/10.1016/S1474-4422(15)00017-4] [PMID: 25908089]

[42]   Derdeyn CP, Chimowitz MI, Lynn MJ, *et al.* Aggressive medical treatment with or without stenting in high-risk patients with intracranial artery stenosis (SAMMPRIS): the final results of a randomised trial. Lancet 2014; 383(9914): 333-41.
[http://dx.doi.org/10.1016/S0140-6736(13)62038-3] [PMID: 24168957]

[43]   Zaidat OO, Fitzsimmons BF, Woodward BK, *et al.* Effect of a balloon-expandable intracranial stent *vs* medical therapy on risk of stroke in patients with symptomatic intracranial stenosis: the VISSIT randomized clinical trial. JAMA 2015; 313(12): 1240-8.

[http://dx.doi.org/10.1001/jama.2015.1693] [PMID: 25803346]

[44]   Esposito G, Amin-Hanjani S, Regli L. Role of and indications for bypass surgery after Carotid Occlusion Surgery Study (COSS)? Stroke 2016; 47(1): 282-90.
[http://dx.doi.org/10.1161/STROKEAHA.115.008220] [PMID: 26658449]

[45]   Endarterectomy for asymptomatic carotid artery stenosis. Executive Committee for the Asymptomatic Carotid Atherosclerosis Study. JAMA 1995; 273(18): 1421-8.
[http://dx.doi.org/10.1001/jama.1995.03520420037035] [PMID: 7723155]

[46]   Hobson RW II, Weiss DG, Fields WS, *et al.* Efficacy of carotid endarterectomy for asymptomatic carotid stenosis. N Engl J Med 1993; 328(4): 221-7.
[http://dx.doi.org/10.1056/NEJM199301283280401] [PMID: 8418401]

[47]   Brott TG, Hobson RW II, Howard G, *et al.* Stenting *versus* endarterectomy for treatment of carotid-artery stenosis. N Engl J Med 2010; 363(1): 11-23.
[http://dx.doi.org/10.1056/NEJMoa0912321] [PMID: 20505173]

[48]   Rosenfield K, Matsumura JS, Chaturvedi S, *et al.* Randomized trial of stent *versus* surgery for asymptomatic carotid stenosis. N Engl J Med 2016; 374(11): 1011-20.
[http://dx.doi.org/10.1056/NEJMoa1515706] [PMID: 26886419]

[49]   Whitty CJ, Sudlow CL, Warlow CP. Investigating individual subjects and screening populations for asymptomatic carotid stenosis can be harmful. J Neurol Neurosurg Psychiatry 1998; 64(5): 619-23.
[http://dx.doi.org/10.1136/jnnp.64.5.619] [PMID: 9598677]

CHAPTER 4

Medical and Surgical Treatment of Stroke

Bruce C.V. Campbell[*] and **Stephen M. Davis**

Department of Medicine and Neurology, Melbourne Brain Centre at The Royal Melbourne Hospital, University of Melbourne, Melbourne, Australia

Abstract: Treatment of stroke patients should occur in dedicated stroke units with experienced medical, nursing and allied health staff to minimize morbidity and mortality. Specific treatment strategies depend on the type of stroke, which is determined by urgent brain imaging. The key treatment for ischaemic stroke, caused by a blocked blood vessel, is to restore blood flow using clot-dissolving medicine or minimally invasive surgery *via* angiogram. Both treatments are time critical as effectiveness reduces rapidly over the first few hours after stroke onset. Specific treatment options for intracerebral haemorrhage (bleeding into the brain) are limited, but lowering blood pressure may have some benefit and research into minimally invasive surgery is ongoing. In addition to lifestyle modification, prevention of further strokes requires lowering blood pressure and, for ischaemic stroke, lowering cholesterol and medications to reduce clotting (*e.g.* aspirin). Access to proven stroke therapies is highly variable and gaps lead to unnecessary disability, death and health costs.

Keywords: Cytoprotection, Intracerebral haemorrhage, Ischaemic stroke, Nanoparticles, Stem cell therapy, Stroke unit, Thrombectomy, Thrombolysis, Virtual rehabilitation.

INTRODUCTION

This chapter addresses the following questions.

1. What basic stroke care elements improve outcomes for a broad range of stroke patients?
2. What strategies that restore blood flow to the brain improve outcomes for ischaemic stroke patients?
3. Does surgical decompression improve outcomes for patients with large ischaemic stroke?
4. What medical interventions improve outcome in intracerebral haemorrhage?
5. What surgical interventions improve outcome in intracerebral haemorrhage?

[*] **Corresponding author Bruce C.V. Campbell:** Department of Neurology, Royal Melbourne Hospital, Parkville VIC 3050, Australia;; Tel/Fax: +61 3 9342 8448/+61 3 9342 8427; E-mail: bruce.campbell@mh.org.au

Shanthi Mendis (Ed.)

6. Do strategies to reduce secondary injury (cytoprotection) improve outcome after stroke?

7. Who should take what action to improve the current situation/ gaps/ inequalities?

1. WHAT BASIC STROKE CARE ELEMENTS IMPROVE OUTCOMES FOR A BROAD RANGE OF STROKE PATIENTS?

Stroke Unit Care

Scientific studies (randomized controlled trials) of organized stroke care in a geographically defined stroke unit have demonstrated important reductions in morbidity (disease course) and mortality (death) compared to general medical care [1]. These benefits apply to all stroke subtypes, severities and demographic subgroups. The precise contributors to this effect are difficult to tease out, but are thought to include medical, nursing and allied health staff with specialist knowledge, interest and experience in managing stroke and preventing complications.

Prevention of aspiration pneumonia (lung infection due to food and oral secretions entering the airways when swallowing) with early swallow safety assessment is a key component. Nursing staff can often make an initial screening assessment of safety when trained with a validated screening tool. Speech therapist expertise can then be reserved for patients who fail screening, often due to the presence of a facial droop or a brainstem stroke that are associated with a higher risk of swallowing difficulties.

Patients with stroke are at high risk of deep venous thrombosis (DVT – clots in the veins of the legs) due to immobility and potentially fatal pulmonary embolism (migration of a clot to the lung where it can cause serious breathing problems and death). The use of pharmacological prevention of deep vein thrombosis (heparin or low molecular weight heparin) is generally recommended for patients with strokes due to blocked cerebral vessels (ischaemic stroke). Mechanical calf compression also has proven beneficial in reducing deep vein thrombosis and is particularly useful in patients with stroke due to bleeding in the brain (intracerebral haemorrhage) and ischaemic stroke patients at higher risk of bleeding complications such as in the first 24 hours after thrombolysis [2].

Early mobilization has been widely espoused, but a recent scientific study (the AVERT trial) demonstrated that ultra-early and intensive mobilization in the first 24 hours can be harmful for some patients [3]. The mechanism of this detrimental effect is not fully elucidated, but applied to both ischaemic stroke and intracerebral haemorrhage.

For some patients, especially those with pre-existing co-morbidities, stroke is their final illness. End-of-life care (palliation or comfort care) is an important component of stroke unit care that contributes to quality of life for patients and relatives.

Secondary Stroke Prevention (Preventing Recurrent Attacks of Stroke)

Those who develop a stroke are prone to repeated attacks of stroke. Appropriate secondary stroke prevention requires investigation for the cause of stroke. Essential investigations in ischaemic stroke include imaging the carotid arteries for strokes affecting that arterial territory and heart rhythm (ECG) monitoring to detect irregular heart rhythms.

Young stroke patients and those without traditional vascular risk factors require more intensive investigation to cover additional causes of stroke such as arterial dissection (a tear in the wall of an artery), which can be imaged with computerized tomography or magnetic resonance angiography, various heart abnormalities that can be screened for with ultrasound imaging (echocardiogram) and blood tests for clotting diseases. Patients with intracerebral haemorrhage should generally have arterial imaging to exclude underlying vessel abnormalities and follow-up imaging to ensure there is no lesion (such as a tumour) underlying the bleed. Venous sinus thrombosis (a clot in the veins draining the brain) also needs to be considered.

Blood Pressure

Blood pressure control is applicable to all stroke subtypes with no evidence of a lower threshold to target [4]. The level of blood pressure reduction appears to be more important than the specific agent used to achieve blood pressure lowering. Recent studies have confirmed observational evidence with blood pressure ~120 mmHg systolic associated with a lower cardiovascular risk than 130 mmHg or 140 mmHg systolic (although patients with a history of stroke were excluded from these studies and stroke itself was not significantly reduced) [5].

Antiplatelets and Anticoagulants

For ischaemic stroke in patients with normal heart rhythm, antiplatelet agents such as aspirin, aspirin-dipyridamole or clopidogrel are proven to reduce recurrent stroke. Combining aspirin and clopidogrel in the short term may be beneficial in high-risk patients [6]. The evidence in support of this came from a large Chinese trial where the diseased vessels were more commonly within the brain rather than in the neck vessels and more frequently affected Western populations. An ongoing trial is investigating short-term aspirin and clopidogrel in Western patients. Long-term combined aspirin and clopidogrel have been shown to increase bleeding risk that offsets any potential stroke prevention benefit. There is evidence that initiating aspirin within the first 48 hours after stroke improves outcomes.

If patients have an irregular heart rhythm, called atrial fibrillation or atrial flutter, then antiplatelet agents are ineffective and anticoagulation is required. Traditionally this was achieved with warfarin, but there are now safer and more effective "direct oral anticoagulants" (DOACs) that are simpler to use for the majority of patients who do not have poor kidney function or mechanical heart valves. Atrial fibrillation is often paroxysmal, which can make it hard to detect. Recent studies using implantable devices that continuously monitor heart rhythm for up to three years have demonstrated ~30% of patients in whom no cause was found for the stroke actually have episodes of atrial fibrillation [7]. This indicates that more thorough search for irregular heart rhythms is necessary.

Cholesterol Lowering

High cholesterol is a weaker risk factor for stroke than it is for heart disease. Nonetheless, intensively lowering cholesterol with "statins" has been shown to improve outcomes in ischaemic stroke [8]. There has been concern that statins may increase the risk of intracerebral haemorrhage although the evidence is equivocal. Statins are not commenced in intracerebral haemorrhage patients, but may be continued if the patient has ischaemic heart disease.

Quitting Tobacco, Engaging in Regular Physical Activity and Consuming a Healthy Diet

Tobacco use is a risk factor for all stroke subtypes and patients are strongly counselled to quit smoking. Several smoking cessation medicines have warnings about use in patients who have had a stroke, but the major benefits of quitting need to be weighed against these theoretical risks. Physical inactivity and obesity are increasingly prevalent and contribute to stroke risk through multiple mechanisms, including high blood pressure, high cholesterol, diabetes and an inflammatory state. Even 30 minutes a day of brisk walking can reduce cardiovascular risk substantially. Calories in the diet should be in balance with energy expenditure to prevent weight gain. Five servings of fruits and vegetables are recommended daily together with restricting salt intake (to less than 5 grams per day), limiting saturated fat intake and eliminating industrial trans fats.

2. WHAT STRATEGIES THAT RESTORE BLOOD FLOW TO THE BRAIN IMPROVE OUTCOMES FOR ISCHAEMIC STROKE PATIENTS?

Ischaemic stroke is caused by a blocked artery that should be supplying the brain with oxygen and glucose. When this occurs, there is some capacity to bypass the occlusion through "collateral" or alternative supply vessels. This is generally not enough to maintain the electrical function of brain cells and so the patient has neurological deficits related to the affected brain region (weakness, numbness, speech disturbance, *etc.*). However, in many cases, the collateral flow can maintain basic cellular functions so that brain tissue can remain viable for a few hours. This potentially salvageable brain is termed "ischaemic penumbra" and is the basis of all proven treatments to restore blood flow and improve outcome [9]. Collateral flow varies substantially between patients depending on the location of the blocked vessel and individual variability in blood vessel networks, hence, the volume and duration of survival for penumbral tissue also varies greatly.

The key to differentiating ischaemic stroke and intracerebral haemorrhage is brain imaging – usually with computerized tomography although rapid magnetic resonance imaging is possible in some centres. Intravenous injection of contrast for computerized tomography angiography or perfusion can demonstrate the blocked blood vessel and abnormal collateral blood flow (Fig. **4.1**).

Intravenous Thrombolysis

The standard approach to achieving reperfusion (restoration of blood flow) is intravenous alteplase or "tissue plasminogen activator" (tPA). This substance is present naturally in humans and is manufactured using recombinant genetic technology. The medicine is delivered as an intravenous infusion over one hour with the dose depending on the patient's weight. tPA activates naturally occurring plasminogen to plasmin, which is an enzyme that breaks down the fibrin strands that hold a clot together.

The first positive clinical trial was the National Institute of Neurological Disorders and Stroke (NINDS) tPA Study Group published in 1995 [10]. Since then, several studies have examined tPA effectiveness and it has been shown to reduce disability when administered within 4.5 hours of stroke onset [11]. This 4.5 hour window is a universal feature of stroke guidelines worldwide although the United States Federal Drug Administration label remains 0–3 hours. However, the magnitude of benefit declines substantially over that 4.5 hour period so earlier treatment is much more effective. The "number needed to treat" to achieve an extra patient with excellent functional outcome using tPA increases from 4.5 within 90 minutes, to 9 between 90 and 180 minutes, and to 14 between 180 and

240 minutes. This is a very potent and cost-effective benefit for patients in comparison to treatments in other fields of medicine.

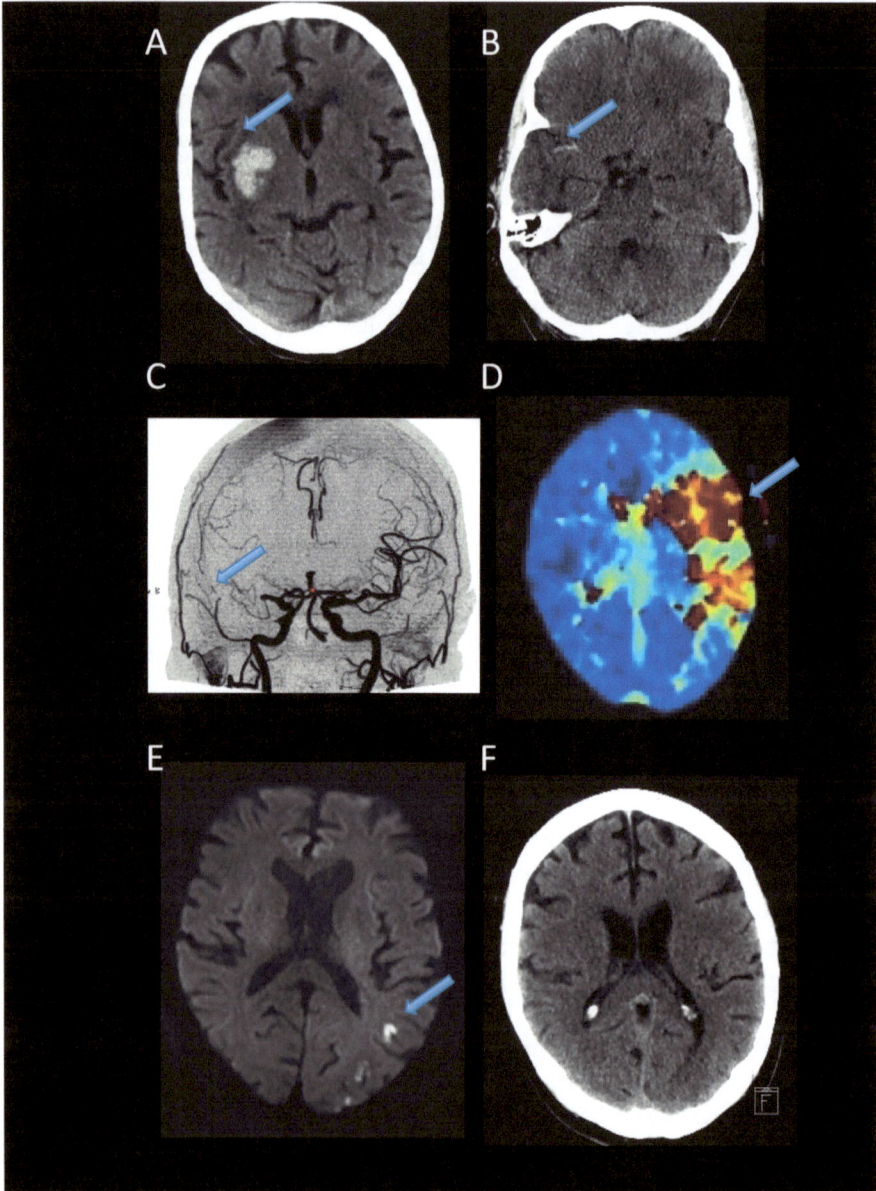

Fig. (4.1). Brain imaging in acute stroke. **A**) CT scan showing intracerebral hemorrhage (arrow). **B**) CT scan showing hyperdense clot in an artery (arrow) and **C**) corresponding blocked artery (arrow) on CT angiogram indicating ischemic stroke. **D**) CT perfusion showing abnormally delayed flow (collateral vessels) diagnostic of ischemic stroke. **E**) MRI diffusion imaging (left) diagnostic of a small ischemic stroke invisible on CT scan (right).

The potential risk of tPA is bleeding. This can occur in the gut or at sites of trauma, but of particular concern is the risk of brain bleeding. Some leakage of blood into an evolving stroke is normal, but development of a significant bleed with pressure effects on surrounding brain can cause clinical deterioration and even death. Symptomatic brain bleeding occurs in ~2% of patients treated with tPA [12]. Patients with more severe strokes affecting larger areas of the brain have a higher risk of brain bleeding. However, tPA has been used for treatment of heart attacks and there was a low rate of brain bleeding even in patients with overtly normal brains (~0.5%).

As experience with tPA has grown, many of the patient groups that were excluded from initial trials have been shown to benefit. In particular, elderly patients were often excluded due to increased rates of poor outcome compared to younger patients in observational series. However, in randomized trials, the treatment benefit in the elderly was at least as great as in younger patients [11]. Confusion between prognostic variables and treatment effect modifiers is a common problem in clinical decision-making. As with most illnesses, elderly patients tend to have worse outcomes than younger patients, but they still do much better with treatment than without it. The individual's functional status is a much more important consideration than their chronological age. Similarly, patients with very severe and very mild stroke have often been excluded from thrombolysis. Severe stroke patients have a worse prognosis, but still derive benefit from treatment. Stroke patients deemed "too mild to treat", usually due to fear of bleeding complication, unfortunately end up with disability in ~30% of cases [13]. The absolute risk of brain bleeding increases with stroke severity so in general the risk–benefit relationship remains proportional. As experience has grown it has become accepted in guidelines that patients taking warfarin anticoagulation can still be safely treated if the level of warfarin activity is relatively low (measured with an INR blood test). Patients with seizure at onset of stroke-like symptoms were excluded in trials due to concern about treating non-stroke mimics, but can now be treated if more advanced brain imaging confirms the presence of a stroke.

Unfortunately, despite having evidence of the efficacy of tPA for over 20 years it remains underutilized. The most active centres deliver tPA to ~20% of their ischaemic stroke patients, but national rates are often ~7%. Given the time dependence of tPA effectiveness the delay from arrival in emergency department to commencing thrombolysis ("door-to-needle" time) is a key determinant of patient benefit. However, many centres still struggle to deliver tPA within 60 minutes of emergency department arrival, despite the best centres having median door-to-needle times under 20 minutes [14, 15]. Simply giving tPA to all eligible patients with best practice door-to-needle times would have major health benefits for communities.

Endovascular Thrombectomy

The concept of inserting a small tube into the arteries of the brain and physically removing a clot has been attempted for decades, but came of age in 2015 with the publication of five positive trials that demonstrated major benefits in reduced disability when this treatment was added to intravenous thrombolysis [16 - 20]. Previous trials published in 2013 failed to demonstrate a benefit, but suffered from earlier generation devices that were relatively ineffective in successfully opening arteries, lack of proof of a target vessel occlusion, delayed treatment and non-consecutive enrolment due to lack of equipoise to randomize all eligible patients [21 - 23]. The positive trials mostly used "stent retriever" devices, whereby a metal cage (stent) is deployed within the clot in the brain artery and then retrieved under suction to capture the clot (Fig. **4.2**).

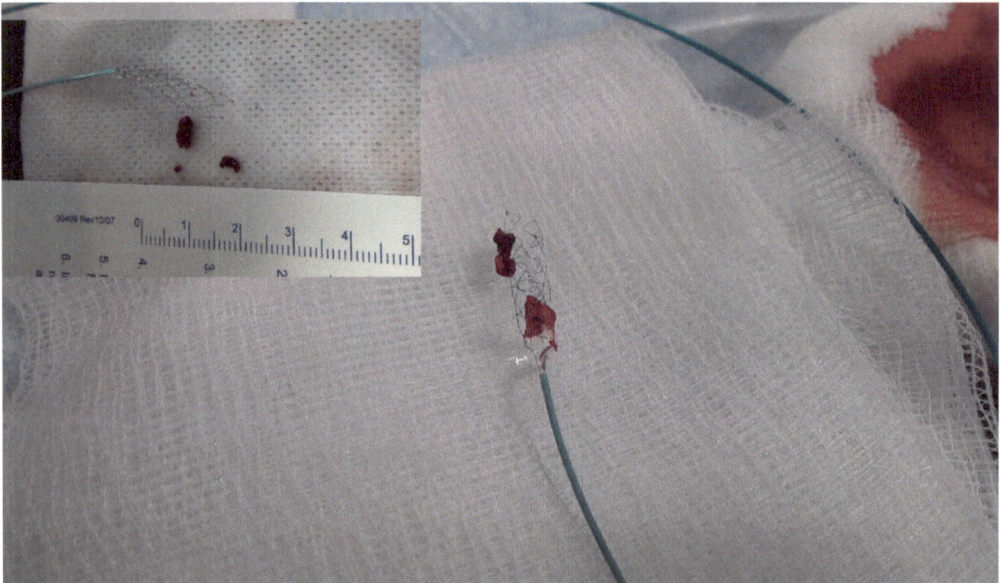

Fig. (4.2). A stent retriever device and retrieved clot.

This technique doubled the rate of successful revascularization compared to the earlier devices. In addition, more advanced brain imaging was used to ensure, at a minimum, that there was indeed a large blocked artery as a target for therapy. Several of the trials also excluded patients with large areas of damaged brain as they were deemed less likely to respond to opening the artery. There was a focus on speed of treatment and the previous neutral trials helped re-establish equipoise and encouraged consecutive recruitment.

An individual patient data meta-analysis from the five trials has been published that addressed many of the questions around subgroups of patients who benefit from endovascular thrombectomy [24]. As with tPA, older patients had poorer outcomes in both intervention and control groups, but there was no evidence of reduced treatment effect in the elderly. Similarly, patients with more severe stroke did not recover as well, but endovascular thrombectomy generated consistently better outcomes across the spectrum of clinical severity. There was no effect of sex and those patients ineligible for intravenous thrombolysis also benefited from endovascular thrombectomy. The treatment benefit was clear cut within six hours of stroke onset. There is evidence from other studies that patients with favourable brain imaging can derive a benefit from restoration of blood flow beyond six hours [25] and several randomized trials are currently exploring this hypothesis.

Endovascular thrombectomy is currently applicable to the larger brain arteries – carotid, basilar and the first part of the middle cerebral artery. Combined occlusions in the neck and brain also benefit. As technology evolves, it may be possible to extend into smaller arteries. However, for now these are best treated with intravenous thrombolysis.

Systems of care are perhaps even more critical for implementation of thrombectomy as the technique requires highly specialized expertise and is, therefore, not available in all hospitals. "Hub and spoke" referral networks are required to rapidly identify and transfer appropriate patients to comprehensive stroke centres. Alternative approaches involving paramedic triage of severe stroke patients likely to have a large vessel occlusion or mobile stroke treatment units equipped with computerized tomography scanners that can positively identify large vessel occlusion in the field are being explored.

Clearly, endovascular thrombectomy is a resource-intensive procedure and will not be applicable in many resource-poor environments. Intravenous thrombolysis will remain the basis of reperfusion therapy in many regions. Potential means to enhance the effectiveness of intravenous thrombolysis with different thrombolytics (*e.g.* tenecteplase [26] and adjunctive strategies are under investigation.

3. DOES SURGICAL DECOMPRESSION IMPROVE OUTCOMES FOR PATIENTS WITH LARGE ISCHAEMIC STROKE?

In addition to the direct injury to brain tissue in the region of stroke, brain swelling can cause secondary injury and death through pressure shifts within the rigid skull compartment. Swelling generally peaks from three to five days after an ischaemic stroke. Younger patients are at greater risk as there is less brain volume loss and, therefore, less space in which to accommodate swelling. In patients with a large hemispheric stroke in the middle cerebral artery territory, the increased swelling can push downwards and cause "coning" with compression of the brainstem where vital heart and breathing functions are controlled, leading to death. A decompressive hemicraniectomy is a neurosurgical procedure that involves removal of a large flap of bone from the skull and cutting the fibrous lining over the brain (dura mater). The bone is stored for later replacement once swelling has resolved. Randomized trials have demonstrated clear benefit of decompressive hemicraniectomy in reducing death and disability in patients with large hemispheric strokes who are under age 60 [27]. Over age 60 it still saves lives, but the degree of disability is high and considerations about desired quality of life need to be weighed [28]. Although many patients prior to stroke state that they would not want to exist in a disabled state, surveys of patients with significant disability following hemicraniectomy generally find that patients, if they had to make the choice again, would still have the surgery.

In the back compartment of the brain, large strokes (ischaemic or intracerebral haemorrhage) affecting the cerebellum can directly compress the vital brainstem or block the passage of cerebrospinal fluid, which causes pressure build-up and coma. Decompression of the posterior fossa – removal of skull and, in this case, often dead brain tissue – is a life-saving procedure. Although there are no randomized trials for this condition, it is generally accepted that the natural history untreated is dire and recovery once the swelling recedes is often excellent.

These procedures are not common and apply to a small minority of stroke patients. Although the evidence for decompressive hemicraniectomy is strong, the practical issue of deciding when to operate is challenging and requires a balance between operating early, when it is not certain that the patient will definitely need decompression, *versus* missing the opportunity by waiting too long with the patient developing irreversible injury as a result.

4. WHAT MEDICAL INTERVENTIONS IMPROVE OUTCOME IN INTRACEREBRAL HAEMORRHAGE?

Intracerebral haemorrhage patients benefit from stroke unit care and mechanical calf compression to reduce the risk of deep vein thrombosis. Beyond these simple measures there is an unfortunate lack of evidence for specific interventions to improve outcome. The bleeding into the brain continues over the first few hours after stroke onset. There is local injury, but pressure effects and shift can also increase disability and cause death.

Intensive Blood Pressure Lowering

The INTERACT and INTERACT-2 studies (Intensive Blood Pressure Reduction in Acute Cerebral Hemorrhage studies) aimed to reduce growth in the volume of bleeding by intensively lowering blood pressure to <140 mmHg systolic (compared to opinion-based guidelines that recommended a target of <180 mmHg). The trials did not show significant reduction in the volume of bleeding, but there was a small magnitude benefit in reduced disability (number needed to treat ~33) [29]. This effect was not replicated in the ATACH2 trial (Antihypertensive Treatment of Acute Cerebral Hemorrhage trial), which used even more intensive targets for blood pressure lowering [30].

Haemostatic Agents to Stop the Bleeding

Given the ongoing growth of the bleed after arrival in hospital, it is attractive to trial medications that promote blood clotting. Recombinant factor VIIa (an activated clotting factor used in haemophiliacs and post-surgical bleeding) was trialled and had promising phase 2 results that failed to replicate in the larger phase 3 trial [31, 32]. Ongoing trials are testing whether this medication can work in a more selected group of patients where continuing bleeding has been demonstrated on a computerized tomography angiogram.

Tranexamic acid has the effect of stabilizing clot formation and has shown a benefit in reducing bleeding complications in major trauma. Ongoing trials are also evaluating tranexamic acid in intracerebral haemorrhage.

5. WHAT SURGICAL INTERVENTIONS IMPROVE OUTCOME IN INTRACEREBRAL HAEMORRHAGE?

Neurosurgical Evacuation

Randomized trials of traditional neurosurgical evacuation, which involves removal of a section of skull and traversing normal brain to access the bleed, have not demonstrated a significant benefit of an early *versus* delayed surgical intervention [33, 34]. However, trials of surgical procedures are challenging and these trials were complicated by crossover between intervention and control arms. Meta-analysis of all available trials does suggest some benefit of surgery, but in general this is reserved as a life-saving procedure in highly selected patients in most Western countries.

Minimally Invasive Clot Evacuation

In parts of Asia, where intracerebral haemorrhage is more common, stereotactic evacuation of the blood clot has been performed although there are no randomized trials. In China, "craniopuncture" with aspiration of the blood clot is sometimes performed by neurologists. The MISTIE (Minimally Invasive Surgery plus rt-PA for Intracerebral Hemorrhage Evacuation) trial programme has been evaluating a strategy of inserting a small catheter into the clot, once it has been established on serial computerized tomography scans that growth in the bleed has ceased. tPA is then instilled into the catheter to dissolve the blood. In the early phase trials this approach appeared to successfully reduce the volume of blood with acceptable safety. A phase 3 trial is in progress.

Intraventricular Bleeding

Sometimes the bleeding extends into the ventricular system where cerebrospinal fluid circulates. This blood can block the normal circulation of fluid and cause increased pressure and coma. The CLEAR 3 randomized trial (Clot Lysis Evaluation of Accelerated Resolution of Intraventricular Hemorrhage trial) showed that inserting a catheter into the blood-filled ventricle and instilling tPA could clear the blood and reduced mortality (but not disability). Further trials to refine this approach are planned.

Bleeding due to Vascular Malformations

When a brain bleed is due to abnormal blood vessels, surgery is often indicated to secure the abnormal vessels and prevent a recurrence. Subarachnoid haemorrhage involves bleeding around the surface of the brain, usually due to a ruptured aneurysm, which is like a bubble on the wall of the artery that can burst. Aneurysms can be secured using endovascular treatment (inserting a catheter into the involved vessel *via* an angiogram and inserting coils of wire that block blood flow into the aneurysm) or neurosurgery where the artery is exposed and a clip placed around the aneurysm to block entry of blood flow. Where both strategies are possible, endovascular treatment is associated with fewer complications.

After the initial phase when raised pressure inside the skull and blockage of the cerebrospinal fluid flow dominate management there is a risk of the brain arteries going into spasm, which can reduce flow and cause further neurological injury. Treatment of this "vasospasm" involves intravenous fluid and raising blood pressure. Endovascular therapy can be useful to pharmacologically or physically dilate the narrowed vessels.

6.   DO STRATEGIES TO REDUCE SECONDARY INJURY (CYTOPROTECTION) IMPROVE OUTCOME AFTER STROKE?

To date, all the effective treatments for ischaemic stroke have involved restoring blood flow. Multiple molecular targets involved in reperfusion injury and cell death have been shown to reduce stroke severity in animal models and yet failed to translate into effective treatments in human trials. There are a number of potential contributors to this problem. Laboratory practices have sometimes suffered from a lack of rigour expected in clinical trials (*e.g.* blinding, randomization). Clinical trials tend to enrol a highly heterogeneous group of patients with a range of stroke subtypes and etiologies compared to the highly controlled animal models. The time windows used in clinical trials have often been longer than in the animal experiments due to pragmatic recruitment considerations. Until recently, high quality, rapid restoration of blood flow was also the exception rather than the rule, in contrast to the current paradigm with endovascular thrombectomy. In the absence of reperfusion it may be difficult for a cytoprotectant to engender indefinite tissue survival.

One creative approach to tackling delays to initiation of therapy was to start treatment in the ambulance. This was demonstrated in the FAST-MAG trial (Field Administration of Stroke Therapy–Magnesium). Although no benefit of magnesium sulphate ($MgSO_4$) was observed, the median onset to treatment of 45 minutes powerfully demonstrated the feasibility of ambulance treatment [35]. With the advent of highly effective endovascular reperfusion there is renewed, albeit cautious, enthusiasm to try once more to develop cytoprotection as a viable therapeutic strategy. Hypothermia is one of the most consistently beneficial treatments in animal models and has the theoretical advantage of simultaneously targeting multiple mechanisms of tissue injury. It also has translated to clinical benefit in improved neurological outcome after cardiac arrest. Ongoing trials are testing different strategies to achieve hypothermia post-stroke with the optimal depth and duration of cooling currently uncertain.

7. WHO SHOULD TAKE WHAT ACTION TO IMPROVE THE CURRENT SITUATION/GAPS /INEQUALITIES?

There are multiple levels of administrative responsibility for different elements of stroke care that differ between countries. Many of the key implementation priorities traverse these layers and jurisdictions, which adds complexity and requires clinical champions to bring the key stakeholders together. In general terms, the potential roles of different organizations are outlined in Table **4.1**.

Key priorities in maximizing the quality of patient outcomes after stroke are access to stroke unit care and optimization of reperfusion therapy delivery systems. Stroke unit care requires cooperation of a multidisciplinary group of clinicians at an individual hospital. Hospital management needs to support the establishment of a geographically defined unit with appropriate allied health staffing levels. However, given the evidence for reduced length of stay and improved outcomes, this should not be problematic. The excitement surrounding advances in reperfusion can be harnessed to drive improvements in stroke unit access as the platform on which reperfusion therapies are built. Ensuring bed management practices that direct all stroke patients to the designated unit and keep them there for the majority of their admission can be more challenging with demand for beds high in most institutions. Ideally, local governments should strategically locate stroke units to ensure optimal population coverage and avoid duplication of services.

Table 4.1. Potential roles of organizations in optimizing stroke care.

Individual stroke units
- ensure policy and procedure in place
- staffing skill-mix and education
- measurement of quality metrics and continuous improvement strategy
Local health districts
- service planning (hub and spoke within immediate network)
Regional government
- ambulance systems
- inter-hospital transport links and service planning (hub and spoke)
- stroke telemedicine services
- monitoring against quality standards
National government
- clinical practice guidelines
- quality standards
- equitable access to prevention and treatment interventions
- protection of the health of the population, including children
International bodies: World Health Organization, World Stroke Organization, human rights movements
- advise on guidelines and quality standards
- advocate for human right to health and health care

Achieving maximum benefit from intravenous thrombolysis and endovascular thrombectomy requires a high level of coordination and, preferably, strategic location of high-volume centralized comprehensive stroke centres, provided this is economically feasible in the local context. In sparsely populated areas, hub and spoke systems are inevitable as low-volume sites will not generate the critical mass to support a neurointerventional service. Very low-volume sites may not even have the critical mass to support onsite expertise to deliver thrombolysis. Telemedicine is increasingly used to overcome this barrier and is highly successful in a range of health systems.

CONCLUDING REMARKS

The former nihilism that nothing could alter the natural history of stroke has been replaced by highly effective treatments that reduce disability after ischemic stroke. This message still needs greater penetrance in the general community to improve stroke recognition and reduce pre-hospital delays.

The current rates of intravenous thrombolysis and endovascular thrombectomy are much lower at a population level than they are in high performing centers and closing that gap poses significant system challenges in providing broad access to treatments in limited resource settings. Availability of treatment is not sufficient – the technology must be embedded in systems that allow rapid treatment as both ischemic stroke and intracerebral hemorrhage progress rapidly in the first few hours after onset. The right patients must be rapidly identified and transported to the appropriate centre to offer the optimal treatment as fast as possible.

Although stent retrievers have transformed the landscape of endovascular thrombectomy, the benchmark for successful revascularization needs to be raised both for completeness and speed. The recent randomized trial evidence and expanding market will hopefully drive innovation to further advance the field.

CONFLICT OF INTEREST

The authors declare no conflict of interest, financial or otherwise.

ACKNOWLEDGEMENTS

Ms AvisAnne Julien is thanked for copy-editing.

REFERENCES

[1]   Langhorne P, Pollock A. Stroke Unit Trialists' Collaboration. What are the components of effective stroke unit care? Age Ageing 2002; 31(5): 365-71.
[http://dx.doi.org/10.1093/ageing/31.5.365] [PMID: 12242199]

[2]   Dennis M, Sandercock P, Reid J, Graham C, Forbes J, Murray G. CLOTS (Clots in Legs Or sTockings after Stroke) Trials Collaboration. Effectiveness of intermittent pneumatic compression in reduction of risk of deep vein thrombosis in patients who have had a stroke (CLOTS 3): a multicentre randomised controlled trial. Lancet 2013; 382(9891): 516-24.
[http://dx.doi.org/10.1016/S0140-6736(13)61050-8] [PMID: 23727163]

[3]   AVERT Trial Collaboration group. Efficacy and safety of very early mobilisation within 24 h of stroke onset (AVERT): a randomised controlled trial. Lancet 2015; 386(9988): 46-55.
[http://dx.doi.org/10.1016/S0140-6736(15)60690-0] [PMID: 25892679]

[4]   Arima H, Chalmers J, Woodward M, *et al.* PROGRESS Collaborative Group. Lower target blood pressures are safe and effective for the prevention of recurrent stroke: the PROGRESS trial. J Hypertens 2006; 24(6): 1201-8.
[http://dx.doi.org/10.1097/01.hjh.0000226212.34055.86] [PMID: 16685221]

[5]   Wright JT Jr, Williamson JD, Whelton PK, *et al.* SPRINT Research Group. A randomized trial of intensive *versus* standard blood-pressure control. N Engl J Med 2015; 373(22): 2103-16.
[http://dx.doi.org/10.1056/NEJMoa1511939] [PMID: 26551272]

[6]   Wang Y, Wang Y, Zhao X, *et al.* CHANCE Investigators. Clopidogrel with aspirin in acute minor stroke or transient ischemic attack. N Engl J Med 2013; 369(1): 11-9.

[http://dx.doi.org/10.1056/NEJMoa1215340] [PMID: 23803136]

[7]   Sanna T, Diener HC, Passman RS, *et al.* CRYSTAL AF Investigators. Cryptogenic stroke and underlying atrial fibrillation. N Engl J Med 2014; 370(26): 2478-86.
[http://dx.doi.org/10.1056/NEJMoa1313600] [PMID: 24963567]

[8]   Amarenco P, Bogousslavsky J, Callahan A III, *et al.* Stroke Prevention by Aggressive Reduction in Cholesterol Levels (SPARCL) Investigators. High-dose atorvastatin after stroke or transient ischemic attack. N Engl J Med 2006; 355(6): 549-59.
[http://dx.doi.org/10.1056/NEJMoa061894] [PMID: 16899775]

[9]   Astrup J, Siesjö BK, Symon L. Thresholds in cerebral ischemia - the ischemic penumbra. Stroke 1981; 12(6): 723-5.
[http://dx.doi.org/10.1161/01.STR.12.6.723] [PMID: 6272455]

[10] National Institute of Neurological Disorders and Stroke rt-PA Stroke Study Group. Tissue plasminogen activator for acute ischemic stroke. N Engl J Med 1995; 333(24): 1581-7.
[http://dx.doi.org/10.1056/NEJM199512143332401] [PMID: 7477192]

[11] Emberson J, Lees KR, Lyden P, *et al.* Stroke Thrombolysis Trialists' Collaborative Group. Effect of treatment delay, age, and stroke severity on the effects of intravenous thrombolysis with alteplase for acute ischaemic stroke: a meta-analysis of individual patient data from randomised trials. Lancet 2014; 384(9958): 1929-35.
[http://dx.doi.org/10.1016/S0140-6736(14)60584-5] [PMID: 25106063]

[12] Wahlgren N, Ahmed N, Dávalos A, *et al.* SITS-MOST investigators. Thrombolysis with alteplase for acute ischaemic stroke in the Safe Implementation of Thrombolysis in Stroke-Monitoring Study (SITS-MOST): an observational study. Lancet 2007; 369(9558): 275-82.
[http://dx.doi.org/10.1016/S0140-6736(07)60149-4] [PMID: 17258667]

[13] Smith EE, Abdullah AR, Petkovska I, Rosenthal E, Koroshetz WJ, Schwamm LH. Poor outcomes in patients who do not receive intravenous tissue plasminogen activator because of mild or improving ischemic stroke. Stroke 2005; 36(11): 2497-9.
[http://dx.doi.org/10.1161/01.STR.0000185798.78817.f3] [PMID: 16210552]

[14] Meretoja A, Strbian D, Mustanoja S, Tatlisumak T, Lindsberg PJ, Kaste M. Reducing in-hospital delay to 20 minutes in stroke thrombolysis. Neurology 2012; 79(4): 306-13.
[http://dx.doi.org/10.1212/WNL.0b013e31825d6011] [PMID: 22622858]

[15] Meretoja A, Weir L, Ugalde M, *et al.* Helsinki model cut stroke thrombolysis delays to 25 minutes in Melbourne in only 4 months. Neurology 2013; 81(12): 1071-6.
[http://dx.doi.org/10.1212/WNL.0b013e3182a4a4d2] [PMID: 23946303]

[16] Berkhemer OA, Fransen PS, Beumer D, *et al.* MR CLEAN Investigators. A randomized trial of intraarterial treatment for acute ischemic stroke. N Engl J Med 2015; 372(1): 11-20.
[http://dx.doi.org/10.1056/NEJMoa1411587] [PMID: 25517348]

[17] Campbell BC, Mitchell PJ, Kleinig TJ, *et al.* EXTEND-IA Investigators. Endovascular therapy for ischemic stroke with perfusion-imaging selection. N Engl J Med 2015; 372(11): 1009-18.
[http://dx.doi.org/10.1056/NEJMoa1414792] [PMID: 25671797]

[18] Goyal M, Demchuk AM, Menon BK, *et al.* ESCAPE Trial Investigators. Randomized assessment of rapid endovascular treatment of ischemic stroke. N Engl J Med 2015; 372(11): 1019-30.
[http://dx.doi.org/10.1056/NEJMoa1414905] [PMID: 25671798]

[19] Jovin TG, Chamorro A, Cobo E, *et al.* REVASCAT Trial Investigators. Thrombectomy within 8 hours after symptom onset in ischemic stroke. N Engl J Med 2015; 372(24): 2296-306.
[http://dx.doi.org/10.1056/NEJMoa1503780] [PMID: 25882510]

[20] Saver JL, Goyal M, Bonafe A, *et al.* SWIFT PRIME Investigators. Stent-retriever thrombectomy after intravenous t-PA *vs.* t-PA alone in stroke. N Engl J Med 2015; 372(24): 2285-95.
[http://dx.doi.org/10.1056/NEJMoa1415061] [PMID: 25882376]

[21]   Broderick JP, Palesch YY, Demchuk AM, *et al.* Interventional Management of Stroke (IMS) III Investigators. Endovascular therapy after intravenous t-PA *versus* t-PA alone for stroke. N Engl J Med 2013; 368(10): 893-903.
[http://dx.doi.org/10.1056/NEJMoa1214300] [PMID: 23390923]

[22]   Ciccone A, Valvassori L, Nichelatti M, *et al.* SYNTHESIS Expansion Investigators. Endovascular treatment for acute ischemic stroke. N Engl J Med 2013; 368(10): 904-13.
[http://dx.doi.org/10.1056/NEJMoa1213701] [PMID: 23387822]

[23]   Kidwell CS, Jahan R, Gornbein J, *et al.* MR RESCUE Investigators. A trial of imaging selection and endovascular treatment for ischemic stroke. N Engl J Med 2013; 368(10): 914-23.
[http://dx.doi.org/10.1056/NEJMoa1212793] [PMID: 23394476]

[24]   Goyal M, Menon BK, van Zwam WH, *et al.* HERMES collaborators. Endovascular thrombectomy after large-vessel ischaemic stroke: a meta-analysis of individual patient data from five randomised trials. Lancet 2016; 387(10029): 1723-31.
[http://dx.doi.org/10.1016/S0140-6736(16)00163-X] [PMID: 26898852]

[25]   Lansberg MG, Cereda CW, Mlynash M, *et al.* Diffusion and Perfusion Imaging Evaluation for Understanding Stroke Evolution 2 (DEFUSE 2) Study Investigators. Response to endovascular reperfusion is not time-dependent in patients with salvageable tissue. Neurology 2015; 85(8): 708-14.
[http://dx.doi.org/10.1212/WNL.0000000000001853] [PMID: 26224727]

[26]   Parsons M, Spratt N, Bivard A, *et al.* A randomized trial of tenecteplase *versus* alteplase for acute ischemic stroke. N Engl J Med 2012; 366(12): 1099-107.
[http://dx.doi.org/10.1056/NEJMoa1109842] [PMID: 22435369]

[27]   Vahedi K, Hofmeijer J, Juettler E, *et al.* DECIMAL, DESTINY, and HAMLET investigators. Early decompressive surgery in malignant infarction of the middle cerebral artery: a pooled analysis of three randomised controlled trials. Lancet Neurol 2007; 6(3): 215-22.
[http://dx.doi.org/10.1016/S1474-4422(07)70036-4] [PMID: 17303527]

[28]   Jüttler E, Unterberg A, Woitzik J, *et al.* DESTINY II Investigators. Hemicraniectomy in older patients with extensive middle-cerebral-artery stroke. N Engl J Med 2014; 370(12): 1091-100.
[http://dx.doi.org/10.1056/NEJMoa1311367] [PMID: 24645942]

[29]   Anderson CS, Chalmers J, Stapf C. Blood-pressure lowering in acute intracerebral hemorrhage. N Engl J Med 2013; 369(13): 1274-5.
[PMID: 24066751]

[30]   Qureshi AI, Palesch YY, Barsan WG, *et al.* ATACH-2 Trial Investigators and the Neurological Emergency Treatment Trials Network. Intensive blood-pressure lowering in patients with acute cerebral hemorrhage. N Engl J Med 2016; 375(11): 1033-43.
[http://dx.doi.org/10.1056/NEJMoa1603460] [PMID: 27276234]

[31]   Mayer SA, Brun NC, Begtrup K, *et al.* FAST Trial Investigators. Efficacy and safety of recombinant activated factor VII for acute intracerebral hemorrhage. N Engl J Med 2008; 358(20): 2127-37.
[http://dx.doi.org/10.1056/NEJMoa0707534] [PMID: 18480205]

[32]   Mayer SA, Brun NC, Begtrup K, *et al.* Recombinant Activated Factor VII Intracerebral Hemorrhage Trial Investigators. Recombinant activated factor VII for acute intracerebral hemorrhage. N Engl J Med 2005; 352(8): 777-85.
[http://dx.doi.org/10.1056/NEJMoa042991] [PMID: 15728810]

[33]   Mendelow AD, Gregson BA, Fernandes HM, *et al.* STICH investigators. Early surgery *versus* initial conservative treatment in patients with spontaneous supratentorial intracerebral haematomas in the International Surgical Trial in Intracerebral Haemorrhage (STICH): a randomised trial. Lancet 2005; 365(9457): 387-97.
[http://dx.doi.org/10.1016/S0140-6736(05)70233-6] [PMID: 15680453]

[34] Vidale S, Bellocchi S, Taborelli A. Surgery for cerebral haemorrhage--STICH II trial. Lancet 2013; 382(9902): 1401-2.
[http://dx.doi.org/10.1016/S0140-6736(13)62211-4] [PMID: 24243130]

[35] Saver JL, Starkman S, Eckstein M, *et al.* FAST-MAG Investigators and Coordinators. Prehospital use of magnesium sulfate as neuroprotection in acute stroke. N Engl J Med 2015; 372(6): 528-36.
[http://dx.doi.org/10.1056/NEJMoa1408827] [PMID: 25651247]

CHAPTER 5

Stroke Care: Stroke Units, New Therapies, Advances and the Future

Jeyaraj D. Pandian[1,*], Akanksha G. William[1], Peter Langhorne[2] and Richard Lindley[3]

[1] *Department of Neurology, Christian Medical College, Ludhiana, Punjab, India*

[2] *Academic Section of Geriatric Medicine, University of Glasgow, Royal Infirmary, Glasgow, Scotland, UK*

[3] *University of Sydney, New South Wales, Australia*

Abstract: Thrombolysis (clot dissolving using medicine) and thrombectomy (clot removal *via* minimally invasive angiogram) are effective acute treatments for ischaemic stroke, but are expensive and time limited. Specialized stroke units are proven to manage stroke-related sequelae and complications effectively. They make stroke treatment quicker, easier and more accessible for a larger number of patients and have specialized staff, predefined protocols and better rehabilitation outcomes. These stroke units have proven benefits in countries that can afford them, but should be extended even to limited-resource settings when possible. Besides thrombolysis, thrombectomy and stroke unit care, ongoing research is exploring medications that may keep brain tissue in the region of a stroke alive for longer (cytoprotection), technological advances such as nanoparticles to increase the penetration of thrombolytic agents into the clot and stem cell therapies, all of which remain to be proven in large-scale randomized controlled trials. As a significant number of patients live with some level of disability, rehabilitation is important. Newer techniques to augment traditional rehabilitation such as robots and computer-based systems and virtual rehabilitation are some of the options currently being actively studied. These are easy to use and have shown positive results in small scale studies, but may be costly.

Keywords: Cost-effectiveness, Disability, Rehabilitation, Stem cell therapy, Stroke units, Thrombectomy, Thrombolysis.

INTRODUCTION

This chapter addresses the following questions.

1. What is the optimal care for stroke patients admitted in hospital?

* **Corresponding author Jeyaraj D. Pandian:** Department of Neurology, Christian Medical College, Ludhiana, Punjab, India; Tel/Fax: +91 161-2220850; E-mail: jeyarajpandian@hotmail.com

2. What are the key components of stroke unit care?
3. What can be done to improve the quality of stroke services?
4. What action needs to be taken and by whom to address gaps in stroke care?
5. Can new technology increase thrombolysis in stroke patients?
6. Can technology be used in stroke rehabilitation?
7. Does stem cell treatment improve stroke outcome?

1. WHAT IS THE OPTIMAL CARE FOR STROKE PATIENTS IN HOSPITAL?

It is important to note that there is incomplete implementation of the key stroke treatments even in the developed countries of the world (Table **5.1**). Treatments such as thrombolysis and thrombectomy are expensive and may not be affordable for limited-resource settings. In countries with more limited financial resources, but with plentiful "human capital", stroke unit care and rehabilitation are likely to be more affordable. In addition, stroke unit care and rehabilitation are applicable to all stroke types, but thrombolysis and thrombectomy only for ischaemic stroke [1]. However, it should be noted that appropriate investment in acute treatments will reduce the requirement of rehabilitation so a balanced approach is required.

Table 5.1. Benefits of different treatment interventions for stroke.

Intervention*	Absolute Benefit (%)	Maximum Proportion Eligible (%)	Number of Extra independent Survivors per Year
Immediate aspirin	1	80	20
Stroke unit	5	80	100
Early community rehabilitation	5	35	44
Thrombolysis	7	20	35
Thrombectomy	25	10	62

* In order of increasing cost, thrombectomy being the most expensive.

In many countries, the standard pathway of care for stroke patients involves admission to hospital for initial assessment, diagnosis, treatment and rehabilitation. The aim of stroke services in hospital should be to provide the care that stroke patients and their families require and in the most efficient, effective, equitable, timely and humane possible manner. Several factors may influence the delivery of stroke care in hospital:

• effectiveness and cost-effectiveness of service design;
• local health-care economy and culture;
• views and needs of different patient groups; and

• resources available.

Stroke Unit

This is the key component of any stroke service and is the centre of stroke care within hospital. Recent publications have also termed these as "essential" stroke services [2]. The various components of stroke units are evidence based.

Primary Stroke Centre

A system of care providing services to a local area (note that recent publications have also termed these as "advanced" stroke services [2].

Comprehensive Stroke Centre

A system of care incorporating the full range of facilities required for regional stroke care in a high-income setting.

2. WHAT ARE THE KEY COMPONENTS OF STROKE UNIT CARE?

The primary objectives of a hospital-based stroke service are outlined in Fig. (**5.1**) and Table **5.2**.

Table 5.2. Objectives of stroke services.

Objectives	Proposed service options
Prompt and accurate assessment and diagnosis	Transport protocols
	Emergency department and hospital protocols
	Stroke centres
	Telemedicine networks
	Rapid access TIA clinics
Specific acute medical and surgical treatment	Stroke centres
	Telemedicine networks
	Stroke units
Identification and assessment of patients' problems	Stroke units
	Stroke centres
	Telemedicine networks
Secondary prevention of further vascular events	Stroke units
	Stroke centres
	Rapid access TIA clinics
General care, including interventions to resolve problems (includes many aspects of rehabilitation)	Stroke units
Terminal care for patients who are unlikely to survive	Stroke units
Hospital discharge and reintegration into the community	Early supported discharge services
	Discharge planning
Long-term care for severely disabled patients	Outpatient rehabilitation services

TIA = transient ischaemic attack.

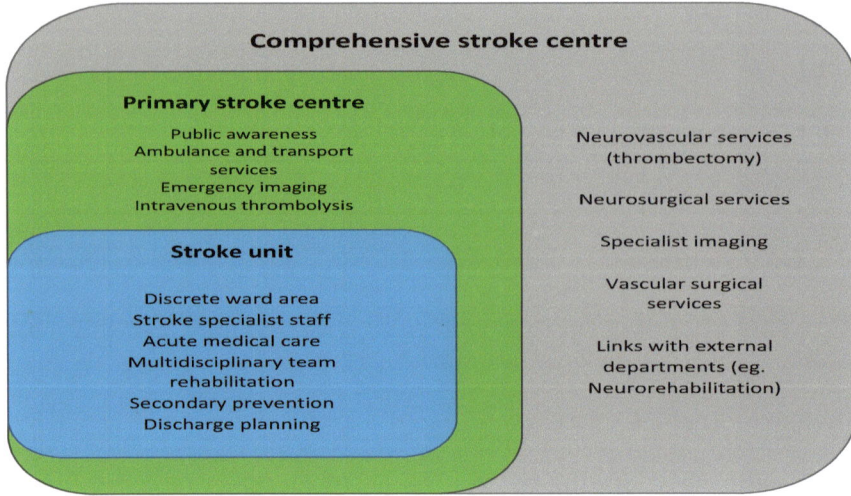

Fig. (5.1). Components of stroke care services.

There are three main reasons why, from an international perspective, the stroke unit should be seen as the central core feature of stroke care and rehabilitation: (i) the population impact is likely to be large [3]; (ii) essential features of care in a stroke unit do not depend on access to high technology facilities and should be widely applicable [3]; and (iii) although it is a complex and multifaceted intervention, the key components are reasonably well described [3, 4] as follows:

- Ward base: Effective stroke units are usually based in a discrete ward with dedicated nursing staff. One of the main advantages of caring for stroke patients in one place is that it can allow the nurses to develop skills to play a major role in the rehabilitation process.
- Specialist staffing: The core medical, nursing and therapy staff should have a specialist interest and expertise in stroke and rehabilitation.
- Acute medical care: Clot retrieval and clot busting therapies are offered to the patient, which are crucial in saving maximum brain tissue. Standard protocols for acute management prevention and treatment of complications and long-term secondary prevention strategies are incorporated in the protocols.
- Multidisciplinary team work: The multidisciplinary team includes a physiotherapist, occupational therapist, speech pathologist, nutritionist, social worker and treating physician. Staff meetings should be held at least once a week to asses and modify the treatment plan of each patient.
- Rehabilitation: The multidisciplinary team therapists assess the stroke patients' functional disability and chart out a treatment plan with short- and long-term goals.

- Secondary prevention: During the stay in a stroke unit, the individual risk factors are identified and appropriate management or surgical treatment is initiated to prevent further stroke.
- Discharge planning: The nurses and physicians plan the discharge after consulting the multidisciplinary team. The patients are either sent home or to a rehabilitation facility.
- Education and training: Regular education and training programmes for stroke care are incorporated in stroke unit care. In addition, patients in stroke care are given sufficient health information regarding prevention of stroke.

Table **5.1** summarizes some of the key processes of care in a stroke unit, including patient assessment, early active management, multidisciplinary rehabilitation and careful discharge planning. There is also an indication that an adapted version of stroke unit care could be widely applied in lower-income settings and further description is found in recent publications [1 - 3].

Stroke Centres

In many wealthy countries, the "essential" stroke unit model of care has been incorporated within a broader and more technological service delivery (Fig. **5.1**), comprehensive stroke centre and primary stroke centre [1]. These services aim to deliver emergency diagnosis and investigations, urgent reperfusion therapies (such as intravenous thrombolysis and mechanical thrombectomy), neurosurgical investigations (*e.g.* decompressive hemicraniectomy), vascular interventions (carotid artery surgery or stenting) and specialist rehabilitation services [1].

3. WHAT CAN BE DONE TO IMPROVE QUALITY OF STROKE SERVICES?

In high-income countries the development of primary stroke centres and comprehensive stroke centres has led to a series of certification programmes [1] and observational studies suggesting an improvement in patient outcomes. Similar approaches and findings have been observed in the delivery of "essential" stroke unit care [5 - 7].

Many stroke services have developed registers to facilitate quality improvement [8]. These approaches have had many features in common and frequently included quality measures to monitor the delivery of care. These quality measures are summarized in Tables **5.3** and **5.4**.

Many such services have undertaken a process of quality improvement that includes:

- identification of key performance indicators;
- definition of recognized standards for these indicators; and
- monitoring of delivery of key performance indicators.

Table 5.3. Features of "essential" stroke unit care.

Patient assessment	Systematic assessment and monitoring of medical, nursing and therapy needs.
Early active management	Management of food and fluids, control of hypoxia, pyrexia and hyperglycaemia plus early mobilization, careful positioning and handling, and avoidance of infection.
Multidisciplinary rehabilitation	Early goal setting with early involvement of caregivers.
Discharge planning	Early planning of needs after discharge.

Table 5.4. Common quality indicators used in stroke registers.

Information collected in the majority of registries	Intravenous thrombolysis Antithrombotic therapy during hospitalization Discharge on antithrombotic medication Management in a stroke unit
Information collected in many registries	Adequacy of fluid and nutrition Assessment of nutritional risk Assessment for swallowing risk Assessment for rehabilitation Imaging (brain or vascular) Carotid endarterectomy or stenting Continence planning Neurosurgery (craniectomy) Discharge on secondary prevention medication Discussion with relative or carer Provision of educational materials Length of stay in hospital Rehabilitation in hospital, including early mobilization Smoking cessation services Team management in stroke unit Time between onset, door, scan and emergency treatment Transport to hospital

Source: Adapted from Cadilhac *et al.* 2016 [8].

Many reports are now available that describe the improvement of services within such processes, particularly in Europe and North America, but they have also been reported in the Far East and Latin America [8]. Some recent research has also demonstrated that the achievement of key performance indicators in routine care is associated with improved patient outcomes such as survival and return home [7].

4. WHAT ACTION NEEDS TO BE TAKEN AND BY WHOM TO ADDRESS GAPS IN STROKE CARE?

Most hospital stroke service improvements are developed through the actions of local "champions". The local champion or head of a stroke unit is usually a physician/neurologist/geriatrician who takes the lead in establishing and running stroke care services. The services offered by all in the multidisciplinary teams are documented in patient charts. In their weekly meetings, progress of patients is discussed and long-term planning of rehabilitation is done. Regular audits are usually incorporated in stroke care services, which helps in looking at gaps in delivery of stroke services.

Health service commissioners, policy-makers and planners need to recognize that stroke is a global/national priority and that there are cost-effective and affordable stroke interventions that require prioritization within national health services, even in resource-constrained settings.

Hospital planners need to recognize the importance of facilitating the development and strengthening of stroke services within their institution. Often this requires reorganization of existing services plus additional investment in more expensive service delivery such as acute treatments. Health-care staff need to be trained and engaged to feel empowered to carry forward service improvements.

5. CAN NEW TECHNOLOGY IMPROVE EFFICACY OF THROMBOLYSIS IN STROKE PATIENTS?

Sonothrombolysis

Ultrasound waves when combined with intravenous (IV) thrombolysis is termed sonothrombolysis (Fig. **5.2**). In this experimental method, waves of 2 MHz are applied during and after administration of clot busting drugs (tPA). These ultrasound waves promote circulation of clot busting drugs, increase the clot surface that is in contact with the drug [9] and reversibly break the crosslinked fibrin fibres (Fig. **5.3**) [10]. Although it is associated with better restoration of the blood flow, it may increase the risk of symptomatic intracerebral haemorrhage [11 - 16]. Adding microbubbles further helps in restoring the blood flow. These microbubbles are made from gasses dissolved in a liquid medium. They are synthesized by mechanical agitation, sonication or the use of microfluidic devices. Their behaviour and movement in the body can be controlled by external ultrasound waves. These waves can agitate these microbubbles (vibrate at a higher frequency), move in a circular fashion and even collapse. All this causes mechanical fragmentation of the clot and clot busting drugs can be delivered further inside the clot [17].

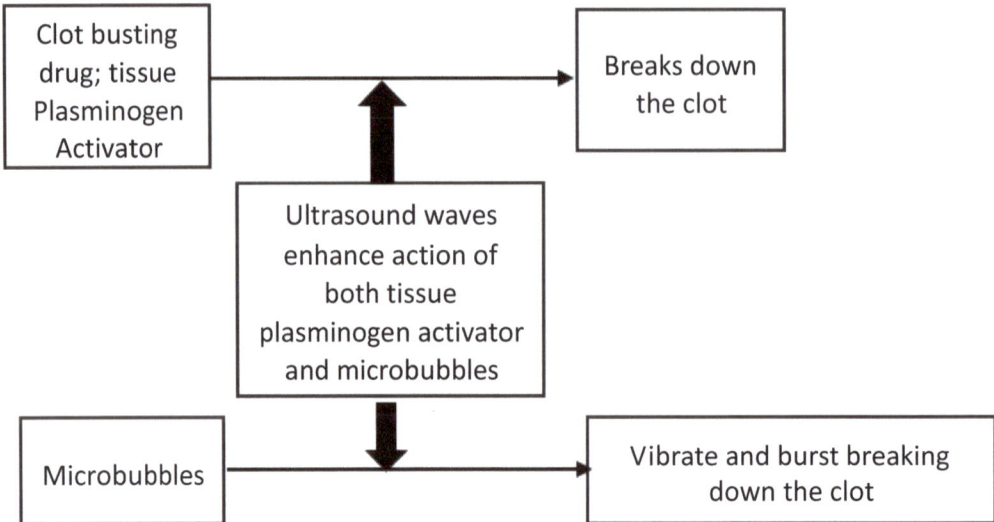

Fig. (5.2).   Shows how ultrasound waves enhance action of both tissue plasminogen activator and microbubbles.

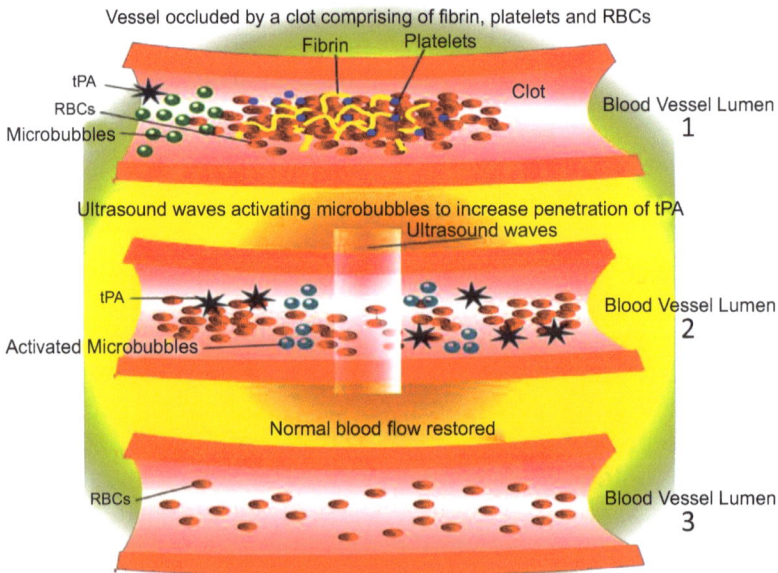

Fig. (5.3).   Microbubble-enhanced sonothrombolysis of occlusive clot.
Notes: The upper most image depicts a vascular occlusion caused by a clot that comprises fibrin, platelets and red blood cells. The second image depicts ultrasound activated microbubbles (*e.g.* by IV injection). The third image depicts blood flow restored to normal.
Design: Dr Vinay Wilson, Department of Neurology, Christian Medical College, Ludhiana, India.

Nanoparticles

As the name suggests, nanoparticles are very small particles that cross the blood brain barrier without compromising its integrity. They can be micelles, inelastic spherical shells, nano-tubular particles, liposomes, golden nanoparticles, *etc*. Their size varies from 1–300 nanometres. Cilostazol nanoparticles have been shown to reduce the infarct area in animal experiments [18 - 20]. Another promising nanoparticle was developed by a team of scientists from Houston Methodist Research Institute, which has an external coating of albumin and contains iron oxide in its core (Fig. **5.4**). External magnetic fields could guide the nanoparticles to the blood clot and localized magnetic heating could speed clot dissolution (Fig. **5.5**). The albumin coating protects it from the human immune system.

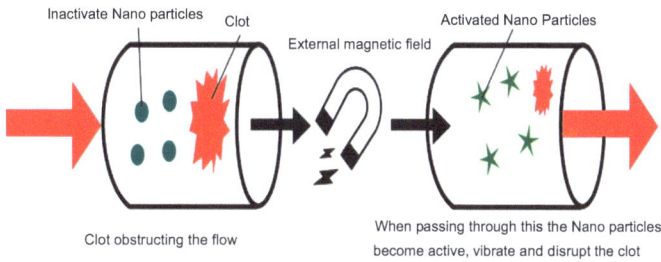

Fig. (5.4). Activation of nanoparticles using external magnetic field; particles vibrate at a greater frequency and bust the clot faster.
Design: Dr Vinay Wilson, Department of Neurology, Christian Medical College, Ludhiana, India.

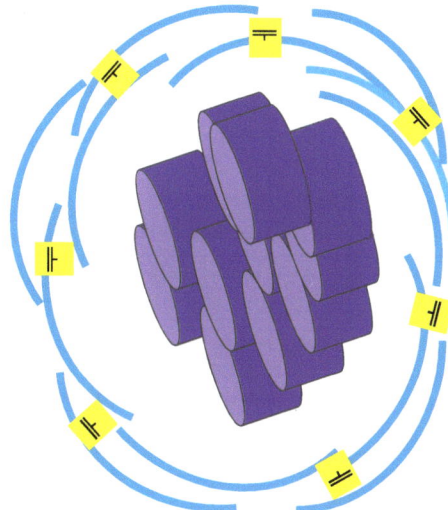

Fig. (5.5). Each nanoparticle is composed of an iron oxide core (purple), surrounded by albumin (blue) and containing tPA (yellow).
Design: Dr Vinay Wilson, Department of Neurology, Christian Medical College, Ludhiana, India.

The administered drug travels around the vascular system, and only some reaches the targeted clot [21]. The reduction in dose means reduced chances of haemorrhage. There is a need for trials to generate evidence of this therapy for stroke. Currently, there is lack of knowledge about drug dosage, decomposition or chemical absorption by the patient's metabolic system [22].

6. CAN TECHNOLOGY BE USED IN STROKE REHABILITATION?

It is important to note that basic rehabilitation is unavailable for many with stroke, and the provision of rehabilitation needs to be a priority for all stroke services. With this proviso, there are exciting new possibilities in this field.

Robotics

These are machines designed to assist or compensate movement. Their ability to be worn externally have made it possible for patients with disability to regain function and for therapy to be offered outside rehabilitation centres. These robots when evaluated for their efficacy are equally effective and sometimes offer greater improvement compared to standard physiotherapy. Rehabilitation robots are of two types:

- End-effector devices – *e.g.* MIT MANUS and Arm guide, which work by applying mechanical forces to the distal segments of limbs. End-effector type robots offer the advantage of easy setup, but suffer from limited control of the proximal joints of the limb, which could result in abnormal movement patterns. These can be programmed to give predefined exercise to the wrist, elbow and shoulder separately and/or simultaneously. Also, these can be programmed to mimic the unimpaired arm in order to provide synchronous exercises.
- Exoskeleton – an external framework strapped on the patient's legs or arms.

There are several commercially available robots, *e.g.* GAITRite, SMAr robots, InMotion Arm Robot (United States) and Armeo Power (Switzerland) (Figs. **5.6** and **5.7**). These robots help by mimicking movements of gait, jumping, stair climbing, *etc* [23].

The Stride Management Assist robotic device developed in Japan is another device. It allows adjustments by a physiotherapist while it is being used and helps in directional stepping, stair climbing and dual tasking among other things. The device weighs 2.8 kilograms and runs on a rechargeable lithium ion battery [23 - 25]. Nearly all trials done to assess the efficacy of robots in rehabilitation concluded that it is beneficial and in some cases superior to conventional therapy. However, they are often heavy, expensive and not readily available. All countries may not have these robots or physiotherapists trained in assisting patients who need them.

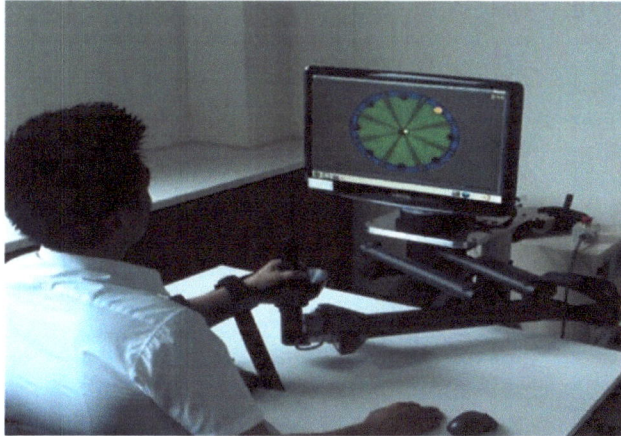

Fig. (5.6). End-effector type – In Motion 2.0 Interactive Motion Technologies, Watertown, MA, USA. Reproduced with permission from *Journal of Stroke*.
Source: Chang WH, Kima YH. Robot assisted therapy in stroke rehabilitation. J Stroke. 2013;15:174–81).

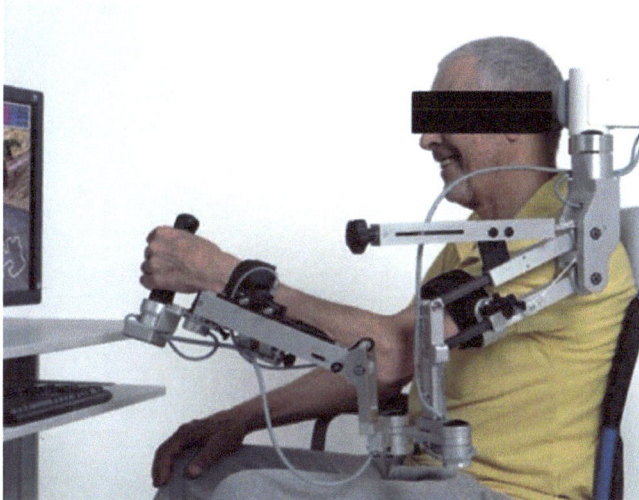

Fig. (5.7). Robotic devices for motor training - Exoskeleton type (Armeo®, Hocoma, Switzerland). Reproduced with permission from *Journal of Stroke*.
Source: Chang WH, Kima YH. Robot assisted therapy in stroke rehabilitation. J Stroke. 2013;15:174–81.

Virtual Rehabilitation

This is a computer-based technology that allows users to interact with a multisensory (visual, auditory and tactile) simulated environment and receive feedback on their performance in a computer-generated scenario (virtual world). This technology is very similar to household videogame systems and involves a hand glove that mimics simple everyday movements, *e.g.* playing checkers, picking up coins and putting them into a bank, putting paper clips onto a piece of paper, tracing geometric designs and eating lunch. Different exercises are designed to focus on different skills, *e.g.* range of motion, speed of movement, fractionation of individual finger motion or strengthening of the fingers (Fig. **5.8**). Some models also have a feedback system that enables comparison of the current performance with that of an earlier one, and hence, can keep a patient motivated [26].

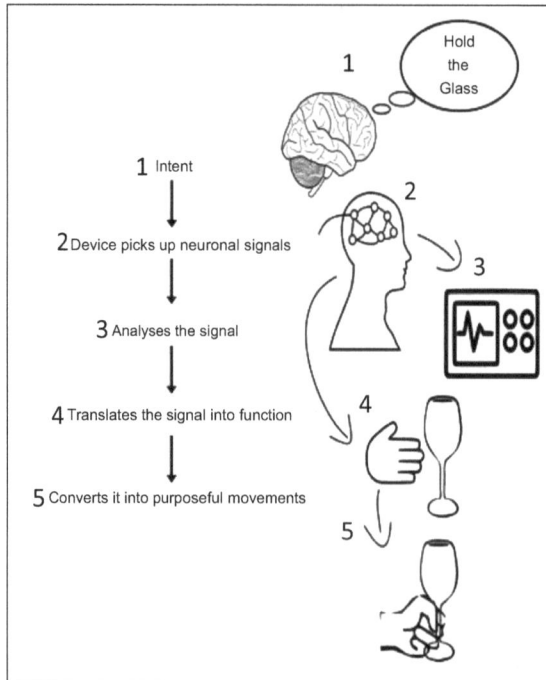

Fig. (5.8). Flow chart depicting conversion of intention to action.
Design: Dr Vinay Wilson, Department of Neurology, Christian Medical College, Ludhiana, India.

Nintendo Wii Gaming System

This is a virtual rehabilitation system that uses a wireless controller to interact with the player through a motion detection system and avatar (computer user's representation of himself or herself or alter ego) technology. This controller uses embedded acceleration sensors responsive to changes in direction, speed and acceleration that enables participants to interact with the games while performing movements using the wrist, arm and hand. An infrared light sensor, on top of a television, captures and reproduces on the screen the movement as performed by participants. The feedback provided by the television screen, as well as the opportunity to observe their own movements in real time, generates positive reinforcement, thus facilitating training and task improvement. Its efficacy has been shown in a trial where it improved mean motor function [27 - 29]. This form of therapy is inexpensive, safe and easy to use for most people.

Brain Computer Interphase

This is a device that responds to neuronal process in the brain and communicates intention to an external device. This technology acquires brain signals, analyses them and translates them into commands that are relayed to output devices that carry out desired actions. The main goal of the device is to restore functionality after disabling neuromuscular disorders such as stroke, spinal injury and amyotrophic lateral sclerosis [30]. If it can be made to control a computer cursor, then the possibilities can be endless for any patient. It is less dependent on residual muscle strength. It was proved feasible in a small clinical study, but trials with more individuals are needed to strengthen the evidence [31]. If moving the impaired limb is difficult and/or impossible even after early participation in an active rehabilitation programme, then this technique can be used to perform repetitions of movement at the cerebral level without any physical activity.

Neuroprotectants

Few neuroprotective agents have been shown to offer benefits in stroke. Citicoline was viewed as a potential neuroprotective agent after numerous trials reported the probability of better recovery. However, a recent meta-analysis involving a large number of patients deduced that it had no beneficial role. Cerebrolysin was another promising neuroprotective agent, but its efficacy is yet to be proven. Trials studying other potential neuroprotective agents have reported little or no benefit [32]. However, some trials offering promising results have been reported in animal models [33].

7. DOES STEM CELL TREATMENT IMPROVE STROKE OUTCOME?

Stem cell therapy is unproven, but offered surprisingly often around the world. It is important that patients and their relatives are not persuaded to buy expensive unproven treatment, while this exciting new treatment is evaluated.

Granulocyte colony stimulating-factor is a cytokine that acts on haematopoietic stem cells and stimulates the growth and survival of neutrophilic granulocyte lineage. It helps in neuronal differentiation, prevents apoptosis, promotes angiogenesis and reduces inflammation. These properties are said to attenuate cerebral ischaemic injury. It is also postulated to generate new neuronal cells.

Meta-analysis from the animal studies suggested that granulocyte colony stimulating-factor both reduces infarct size and enhances functional recovery; in addition, its effect is presumably dose dependent [34]. Subsequent clinical trials were planned to study its effects on humans. A small trial conducted in India on 10 patients did not demonstrate any efficacy, but established its safety, feasibility and tolerability [35]. A study on 58 patients in a multicentric study from India also demonstrated safety, but not efficacy [36]. A recent trial conducted on 18 patients at Stanford University proved that bone marrow-derived mesenchymal stem cells can be used to improve clinical outcome of stroke patients [37].

Researchers at King's College London have developed a technology to harvest neural stem cells that have the potential to be used for stroke. This procedure is called "conditional immortalization", which means that the cell multiplies to yield its exact copies. This will enable offering multiple doses. The technique is still under animal studies with promising results. It was tested in the United Kingdom's first such clinical trial where it was proven safe and, as a result, a phase II clinical trial is actively recruiting patients [38, 39]. Other promising stem cell trials are recruiting patients in other countries [40], while some therapies are also offered on a commercial basis [41, 42].

CONCLUDING REMARKS

There has been a rapid advance in the treatment of acute stroke in the form of thrombolysis, thrombectomy and post stroke care services and rehabilitation. Nanoparticle drug delivery systems are being tried to enhance the clot lysis by tPA. Robotic technology, brain computer interface and virtual game systems could provide important augmentation of rehabilitation, and help overcome the shortage of trained local stroke professionals. Stem cell therapy in the acute and chronic phase of stroke are promising, but need to be proved in large-scale trials.

CONFLICT OF INTEREST

The authors declare no conflict of interest, financial or otherwise.

ACKNOWLEDGEMENTS

Ms AvisAnne Julien is thanked for copy-editing.

REFERENCES

[1]   Ringelstein EB, Chamorro A, Kaste M, *et al.* ESO Stroke Unit Certification Committee. European Stroke Organisation recommendations to establish a stroke unit and stroke center. Stroke 2013; 44(3): 828-40.
       [http://dx.doi.org/10.1161/STROKEAHA.112.670430] [PMID: 23362084]

[2]   Lindsay P, Furie KL, Davis SM, Donnan GA, Norrving B. World Stroke Organization global stroke

services guidelines and action plan. Int J Stroke 2014; 9(Suppl. A100): 4-13.
[http://dx.doi.org/10.1111/ijs.12371]

[3]   Langhorne P, de Villiers L, Pandian JD. Applicability of stroke-unit care to low-income and middle-income countries. Lancet Neurol 2012; 11(4): 341-8.
[http://dx.doi.org/10.1016/S1474-4422(12)70024-8] [PMID: 22441195]

[4]   WSO module, reference Available at: http://world-stroke-academy.org/wso/#!*menu=16*browseby=6*sortby=1*label=5943

[5]   Terént A, Asplund K, Farahmand B, *et al.* Stroke unit care revisited: who benefits the most? A cohort study of 105,043 patients in Riks-Stroke, the Swedish Stroke Register. J Neurol Neurosurg Psychiatry 2009; 80(8): 881-7.
[http://dx.doi.org/10.1136/jnnp.2008.169102] [PMID: 19332423]

[6]   Meretoja A, Roine RO, Kaste M, *et al.* Effectiveness of primary and comprehensive stroke centers: PERFECT stroke: a nationwide observational study from Finland. Stroke 2010; 41(6): 1102-7.
[http://dx.doi.org/10.1161/STROKEAHA.109.577718] [PMID: 20395609]

[7]   Turner M, Barber M, Dodds H, Dennis M, Langhorne P, Macleod MJ. The impact of stroke unit care on outcome in a Scottish stroke population, taking into account case mix and selection bias. J Neurol Neurosurg Psychiatry 2015; 86(3): 314-8.
[http://dx.doi.org/10.1136/jnnp-2013-307478] [PMID: 24966391]

[8]   Cadilhac DA, Kim J, Lannin NA, *et al.* National stroke registries for monitoring and improving the quality of hospital care: A systematic review. Int J Stroke 2016; 11(1): 28-40.
[http://dx.doi.org/10.1177/1747493015607523] [PMID: 26763018]

[9]   Polak JF. Ultrasound energy and the dissolution of thrombus. N Engl J Med 2004; 351(21): 2154-5.
[http://dx.doi.org/10.1056/NEJMp048249] [PMID: 15548774]

[10]   Braaten JV, Goss RA, Francis CW. Ultrasound reversibly disaggregates fibrin fibers. Thromb Haemost 1997; 78(3): 1063-8.
[PMID: 9308755]

[11]   Barlinn K, Tsivgoulis G, Barreto AD, *et al.* Outcomes following sonothrombolysis in severe acute ischemic stroke: subgroup analysis of the CLOTBUST trial. Int J Stroke 2014; 9(8): 1006-10.
[http://dx.doi.org/10.1111/ijs.12340] [PMID: 25079049]

[12]   Barreto AD, Alexandrov AV, Shen L, *et al.* CLOTBUST-Hands Free: pilot safety study of a novel operator-independent ultrasound device in patients with acute ischemic stroke. Stroke 2013; 44(12): 3376-81.
[http://dx.doi.org/10.1161/STROKEAHA.113.002713] [PMID: 24159060]

[13]   Tsivgoulis G, Eggers J, Ribo M, *et al.* Safety and efficacy of ultrasound-enhanced thrombolysis: a comprehensive review and meta-analysis of randomized and nonrandomized studies. Stroke 2010; 41(2): 280-7.
[http://dx.doi.org/10.1161/STROKEAHA.109.563304] [PMID: 20044531]

[14]   Ricci S, Dinia L, Del Sette M, *et al.* Sonothrombolysis for acute ischaemic stroke. Cochrane Database Syst Rev 2012; (6): CD008348.
[PMID: 22696378]

[15]   Saqqur M, Tsivgoulis G, Nicoli F, *et al.* The role of sonolysis and sonothrombolysis in acute ischemic stroke: a systematic review and meta-analysis of randomized controlled trials and case-control studies. J Neuroimaging 2014; 24(3): 209-20.
[http://dx.doi.org/10.1111/jon.12026] [PMID: 23607713]

[16]   Bor-Seng-Shu E, Nogueira RdeC, Figueiredo EG, Evaristo EF, Conforto AB, Teixeira MJ. Sonothrombolysis for acute ischemic stroke: a systematic review of randomized controlled trials. Neurosurg Focus 2012; 32(1): E5.
[http://dx.doi.org/10.3171/2011.10.FOCUS11251] [PMID: 22208898]

[17] Zhou XB, Qin H, Li J, *et al.* Platelet-targeted microbubbles inhibit re-occlusion after thrombolysis with transcutaneous ultrasound and microbubbles. Ultrasonics 2011; 51(3): 270-4.
[http://dx.doi.org/10.1016/j.ultras.2010.09.001] [PMID: 20888024]

[18] Panagiotou S, Saha S. Therapeutic benefits of nanoparticles in stroke. Front Neurosci 2015; 9: 182.
[http://dx.doi.org/10.3389/fnins.2015.00182] [PMID: 26041986]

[19] Nagai N, Yoshioka C, Ito Y, Funakami Y, Nishikawa H, Kawabata A. Intravenous administration of cilostazol nanoparticles ameliorates acute ischemic stroke in a cerebral ischemia/reperfusion-induced injury model. Int J Mol Sci 2015; 16(12): 29329-44.
[http://dx.doi.org/10.3390/ijms161226166] [PMID: 26690139]

[20] Cheng R, Huang W, Huang L, *et al.* Acceleration of tissue plasminogen activator-mediated thrombolysis by magnetically powered nanomotors. ACS Nano 2014; 8(8): 7746-54.
[http://dx.doi.org/10.1021/nn5029955] [PMID: 25006696]

[21] Voros E, Cho M, Ramirez M, Palange AL, De Rosa E, Key J, *et al.* TPA immobilization on iron oxide nanocubes and localized magnetic hyperthermia accelerate blood clot lysis. Adv Funct Mater 2015; 25: 1709-18.
[http://dx.doi.org/10.1002/adfm.201404354]

[22] Varna M, Juenet M, Bayles R, Mazighi M, Chauvierre C, Letourneur D. Nanomedicine as a strategy to fight thrombotic diseases. Future Sci OA , 20151(4) [12 June 2016]; Available at: http://www.future-science.com/doi/full/10.4155/fso.15.46
[http://dx.doi.org/10.4155/fso.15.46]

[23] Buesing C, Fisch G, O'Donnell M, *et al.* Effects of a wearable exoskeleton stride management assist system (SMA®) on spatiotemporal gait characteristics in individuals after stroke: a randomized controlled trial. J Neuro Engineering Rehabil , 201512 [8 June 2016]; Available at: http://www.ncbi.nlm.nih.gov/pmc/articles/PMC4545867/

[24] Mehrholz J, Hädrich A, Platz T, Kugler J, Pohl M. Electromechanical and robot-assisted arm training for improving generic activities of daily living, arm function, and arm muscle strength after stroke. Cochrane Database Syst Rev 2012; (6): CD006876.
[PMID: 22696362]

[25] Hsieh YW, Wu CY, Lin KC, Yao G, Wu KY, Chang YJ. Dose-response relationship of robot-assisted stroke motor rehabilitation: the impact of initial motor status. Stroke 2012; 43(10): 2729-34.
[http://dx.doi.org/10.1161/STROKEAHA.112.658807] [PMID: 22895994]

[26] Merians AS, Jack D, Boian R, *et al.* Virtual reality-augmented rehabilitation for patients following stroke. Phys Ther 2002; 82(9): 898-915.
[PMID: 12201804]

[27] Saposnik G, Teasell R, Mamdani M, *et al.* Effectiveness of virtual reality using Wii gaming technology in stroke rehabilitation: a pilot randomized clinical trial and proof of principle. Stroke 2010; 41(7): 1477-84.
[http://dx.doi.org/10.1161/STROKEAHA.110.584979] [PMID: 20508185]

[28] Mouawad MR, Doust CG, Max MD, McNulty PA. Wii-based movement therapy to promote improved upper extremity function post-stroke: a pilot study. J Rehabil Med 2011; 43(6): 527-33.
[http://dx.doi.org/10.2340/16501977-0816] [PMID: 21533334]

[29] Bower KJ, Louie J, Landesrocha Y, Seedy P, Gorelik A, Bernhardt J. Clinical feasibility of interactive motion-controlled games for stroke rehabilitation. J Neuroeng Rehabil 2015; 12: 63.
[http://dx.doi.org/10.1186/s12984-015-0057-x] [PMID: 26233677]

[30] Shih JJ, Krusienski DJ, Wolpaw JR. Brain-computer interfaces in medicine. Mayo Clin Proc 2012; 87(3): 268-79.
[http://dx.doi.org/10.1016/j.mayocp.2011.12.008] [PMID: 22325364]

[31] Ang KK, Guan C. Brain-computer interface in stroke rehabilitation. J Comput Sci Eng 2013; 7: 139-

46.
[http://dx.doi.org/10.5626/JCSE.2013.7.2.139] [PMID: 25120465]

[32]   Majid A, Majid A. Neuroprotection in stroke: past, present, and future. Int Sch Res 2014; 2014: e515716.
[http://dx.doi.org/10.1155/2014/515716]

[33]   Fluri F, Grünstein D, Cam E, *et al.* Fullerenols and glucosamine fullerenes reduce infarct volume and cerebral inflammation after ischemic stroke in normotensive and hypertensive rats. Exp Neurol 2015; 265: 142-51.
[http://dx.doi.org/10.1016/j.expneurol.2015.01.005] [PMID: 25625851]

[34]   Minnerup J, Heidrich J, Wellmann J, Rogalewski A, Schneider A, Schäbitz W-R. Meta-analysis of the efficacy of granulocyte-colony stimulating factor in animal models of focal cerebral ischemia. Stroke 2008; 39(6): 1855-61.
[http://dx.doi.org/10.1161/STROKEAHA.107.506816] [PMID: 18403735]

[35]   Prasad K, Kumar A, Sahu JK, *et al.* Mobilization of stem cells using G-CSF for acute ischemic stroke: a randomized controlled, pilot study, mobilization of stem cells using G-CSF for acute ischemic stroke: a randomized controlled, pilot study. Stroke Res Treat 2011; 2011: 283473.
[http://dx.doi.org/10.4061/2011/283473] [PMID: 22007348]

[36]   Prasad K, Sharma A, Garg A, *et al.* Intravenous autologous bone marrow mononuclear stem cell therapy for ischemic stroke: a multicentric, randomized trial. Stroke 2014; 45(12): 3618-24.
[http://dx.doi.org/10.1161/STROKEAHA.114.007028] [PMID: 25378424]

[37]   Steinberg GK, Kondziolka D, Wechsler LR, *et al.* Clinical outcomes of transplanted modified bone marrow-derived mesenchymal stem cells in stroke: a phase 1/2a study. Stroke 2016. pii:STROKEAHA.116.012995 [Epub ahead of print]

[38]   King's College London - Stem cell therapy to repair stroke damage, [13 June 2016]. Available at: http://www.kcl.ac.uk/ioppn/about/difference/15-Stem-cell-therapy-to-repair-stroke-damage.aspx

[39]   Pilot Investigation of Stem Cells in Stroke Phase II Efficacy (full text view: ClinicalTrialsgov), [13 June 2016]. Available at: https://clinicaltrials.gov/ct2/show/NCT02117635

[40]   Stroke - Stem Cells Australia, [13 June 2016]. Available at: http://www.stemcellsaustralia. edu.au/About-Stem-Cells/Stem-Cell-Clinical-Trials/Neurological-conditions/Stroke.aspx

[41]   Swiss medica clinics, [13 June 2016]. Available at: http://www.startstemcells.com/ swiss-medic--clinics.html

[42]   Prasad K, Mohanty S, Bhatia R, *et al.* Autologous intravenous bone marrow mononuclear cell therapy for patients with subacute ischaemic stroke: a pilot study. Indian J Med Res 2012; 136(2): 221-8.
[PMID: 22960888]

CHAPTER 6

Sustainable Development Goals and Stroke

Shanthi Mendis[*]

Geneva Learning Foundation, Former Senior Adviser, World Health Organization, Geneva, Switzerland

Abstract: The 2030 Agenda for Sustainable Development is an ambitious initiative of the United Nations, with 17 goals and 169 targets, integrating health, economic development, elimination of extreme poverty, social inclusion, environmental sustainability and good governance. The 17 Sustainable Development Goals focus on: poverty; hunger; health education; gender equality; water and sanitation; energy; economic growth and employment; industry, innovation and infrastructure; inequality; sustainable cities; consumption and production; climate change; marine resources; terrestrial ecosystems; peace, justice and accountability; and global partnership for sustainable development. There is a mutually reinforcing relationship between health and the three dimensions of sustainable development – social, economic and environmental. The connectors are health systems, behavioural, biochemical and environmental risk factors, ecosystems and the social and structural determinants of health, including enabling legal environments, financing and governance. In recognition of the negative impact of NCDs including stroke on development, they have been specifically incorporated in Goal 3 of the Sustainable Development Goals. Goal 3 addresses all major health priorities, including stroke and other NCDs, integral for the attainment of the Sustainable Development Goals. The 2030 Agenda for Sustainable Development, integrating health with economic, social and environmental dimensions of development, offers an unprecedented opportunity to address stroke (NCDs) and their determinants through multisectoral and multidimensional approaches.

Keywords: Accountability, Climate change, Consumption and production, Education, Employment, Energy, Gender equality, Health, Industry, Inequality, Infrastructure, Innovation, Justice, Marine resources, Millennium Development Goals, Noncommunicable diseases, Peace, Poverty, Stroke, Sustainable Development Goals, Sustainable cities, Terrestrial ecosystems, Water and sanitation, economic growth, hunger.

[*] **Corresponding author Shanthi Mendis:** Geneva Learning Foundation, Geneva, Switzerland; Tel/Fax: 0041227880311; E-mail: prof.shanthi.mendis@gmail.com

INTRODUCTION

This chapter addresses the following questions.

1. What are the health-related Millennium Development Goals (MDGs)?
2. What is the 2030 Sustainable Development Agenda?
3. How are the Sustainable Development Goals linked to health and stroke (noncommunicable diseases)?
4. What are the 17 Sustainable Development Goals and 169 targets?

1. WHAT ARE THE HEALTH-RELATED MILLENNIUM DEVELOPMENT GOALS?

The eight Millennium Development Goals (MDGs), adopted in 2000, included three health-related goals: reduction in child mortality (Goal 4); reduction in maternal mortality and access to reproductive health care (Goal 5); and reversing the spread of HIV/AIDS, tuberculosis and malaria (Goal 6) [1]. These were instrumental in focusing global attention, development aid and national policies and resources in low- and middle-income countries on these important health issues [2, 3]. By 2015, unprecedented gains were made in combating malaria and tuberculosis, and providing access to antiretroviral medicines [4]. Although gaps remain in access to antenatal care and skilled birth attendance, in some parts of the world, considerable progress was made in the reduction of preventable infant and maternal mortality [4]. NCDs, (including stroke), were not included in the Millennium Development Goals and, therefore, received little global and national attention. In early 2000, bilateral aid for tackling NCDs dropped [5] despite their burgeoning contribution to the burden of global disease.

2. WHAT ARE THE SUSTAINABLE DEVELOPMENT GOALS (SDGS)?

The 2030 Agenda for Sustainable Development has merged the unfinished tasks of the Millennium Development Goals with the Agenda articulated in the 2012 United Nations Conference on Sustainable Development [5, 6]. It is an ambitious Agenda with 17 goals and 169 targets, integrating health, economic development, elimination of extreme poverty, social inclusion, environmental sustainability and good governance. While the Millennium Development Goals focused on low-income countries, the 2030 Agenda for Sustainable Development is universal and relevant to the whole world. The brief outline below on the Sustainable Development Goals and targets is based on information and data obtained mainly from United Nations documents.

3. HOW ARE THE SUSTAINABLE DEVELOPMENT GOALS LINKED TO HEALTH AND STROKE (NONCOMMUNICABLE DISEASES)?

The right to health is the most important fundamental human right [7]. According to the WHO definition: "Health is a state of complete physical, mental and social well-being and not merely the absence of disease or infirmity". There is a reciprocal reinforcing relationship between health and all three aspects of sustainable development – social, economic and environmental. Action on the social and environmental determinants of health is in turn critical to creating inclusive, peaceful, equitable, economically productive and healthy societies [8]. The 2030 Agenda for Sustainable Development is based on this broader notion, extending it to incorporate other species, ecosystems and health risks. The health status of people is dependent on the wide-ranging and interlinked impact of social, economic, behavioural and environmental determinants, including biodiversity and ecosystems. The connectors are health systems, behavioural, biochemical and environmental risk factors, ecosystems and the social and structural determinants of health, including enabling legal environments, financing and governance [8].

The 2030 Agenda for Sustainable Development offers an unprecedented opportunity to address prevention and control of stroke (NCDs) from a multisectoral platform. In this context, to implement policies to effectively address stroke (NCDs), three strategic moves are required. First, governments need to reframe prevention and control of stroke (NCDs) from the disease model to embrace the multisectoral prevention model that underpins the 2030 Agenda for Sustainable Development. Second, health policy-makers need to emphasize and insist on health and health equity in all relevant policies of the agenda. The health sector needs to support and collaborate with other sectors to develop and implement policies and programmes in a way that optimizes co-benefits for all sectors involved [8, 9]. Third, health advocates need to engage with global governance structures to finance and implement the Sustainable Development Goals, including Goal 3 for health. The broad and interlinked nature of the Sustainable Development Goals make this repositioning more practical, feasible and indeed necessary.

4. WHAT ARE THE 17 SUSTAINABLE DEVELOPMENT GOALS AND 169 TARGETS?

4.1. Sustainable Development Goal 1

Sustainable Development Goal 1 calls for an end to poverty in all its forms by 2030. The international poverty line is currently defined at US$ 1.90 or below per person per day. In 2012, about 13% of the world's population was living below the poverty line [10]. If current growth rates prevail for the next two decades, the global poverty rate is expected to fall around 6% in the next 20 years. To eliminate poverty, the poor and vulnerable need to be provided opportunities and access to social protection programmes including social and food assistance, child and maternity benefit programmes as well as social insurance and labour market schemes.

According to United Nations data sources, currently, most poor people in the world do not have access to social protection schemes. In low-income countries, only one out of five poor persons receive any type of social protection [10, 11]. Coverage is better in middle-income countries with two out of three receiving social protection in upper-middle-income countries. The coverage gap is particularly wide in Southern Asia and sub-Saharan Africa.

Table 6.1. Sustainable Development Goal 1 targets.

1.1
By 2030, eradicate extreme poverty for all people everywhere, currently measured as people living on less than US$ 1.25 a day.
1.2
By 2030, reduce at least by half the proportion of men, women and children of all ages living in poverty in all its dimensions according to national definitions.
1.3
Implement nationally appropriate social protection systems and measures for all, including floors, and by 2030 achieve substantial coverage of the poor and the vulnerable.
1.4
By 2030, ensure that all men and women, in particular the poor and the vulnerable, have equal rights to economic resources, as well as access to basic services, ownership and control over land and other forms of property, inheritance, natural resources, appropriate new technology and financial services, including microfinance.
1.5
By 2030, build the resilience of the poor and those in vulnerable situations and reduce their exposure and vulnerability to climate-related extreme events and other economic, social and environmental shocks and disasters.
1.a
Ensure significant mobilization of resources from a variety of sources, including through enhanced development cooperation, in order to provide adequate and predictable means for developing countries, in particular least-developed countries, to implement programmes and policies to end poverty in all its dimensions.
1.b
Create sound policy frameworks at the national, regional and international levels, based on pro-poor and gender-sensitive development strategies, to support accelerated investment in poverty eradication actions.

Source: United Nations. Sustainable Development Goals Knowledge Platform.
https://sustainabledevelopment.un.org

Poverty is a predisposing factor for stroke. Poverty also worsens the outcomes of stroke. Poverty leads to poor health literacy, high rates of tobacco use and harmful use of alcohol, poor diet, increased socioeconomic stress, inadequate access to health care services and poor adherence to prevention approaches, and late diagnosis of hypertension and diabetes mellitus, which predispose to stroke and worsen the outcomes [12, 13]. Most stroke centres in low- and middle-income countries are currently in the private sector where fees are levied for services [14]. The poor often lack access to medical care and many treatment options for acute stroke are unaffordable to the poor, resulting in high case fatality rates [15]. Well-organized stroke services and emergency transport services are not available in under-developed areas of developing countries [16]. Up to 84% of stroke patients in developing countries (*versus* 16% in high income countries) die within three years of diagnosis. Furthermore, epidemiological data from the poorest countries reveal a predominance of nonatherosclerotic stroke due to high rates of rheumatic heart valve lesions, a disease directly linked to poverty [17]. Actions to attain the targets of this goal, listed in Table **6.1**, will help to reduce inequities related to stroke occurrence and outcomes of stroke [13].

4.2. Sustainable Development Goal 2

Sustainable Development Goal 2 aims to end hunger and all forms of malnutrition by 2030 (Table **6.2**). Most of the countries that did not reach the target set as part of the Millennium Development Goals of halving the proportion of people who suffer from hunger have faced natural and human-induced disasters or political volatility. According to United Nations data sources, globally, the prevalence of hunger has declined, and is at 11% [10, 11]. However, if current trends continue, the zero hunger target is unlikely to be attained by 2030. Worldwide in 2014, an estimated total of 159 million children had stunted growth. Southern Asia and sub-Saharan Africa accounted for the majority (75%) of the children under 5 with stunted growth.

Another concern related to child nutrition is the growing share of children who are overweight or obese, a risk factor directly related to stroke, diabetes and other NCDs. Globally, in 2015 the number of overweight children under 5 was estimated at over 42 million [18]. Almost 75% of them lived in Africa and Asia. Overweight and obese children are likely to continue to be obese into adulthood. They are more likely to develop diabetes, stroke and heart disease at a younger age. The rise in childhood overweight and obesity are mainly due to a global shift in diet towards increased intake of energy-rich foods coupled with a trend towards decreased physical activity.

Early life nutritional conditions have been shown to impact on risk of developing adult-onset disorders such as stroke and NCDs [19 - 21]. Studies on low-birt--weight cohorts demonstrate that maternal, fetal, neonatal and early life malnutrition increase the risk of hypertension and diabetes in adulthood [19 - 21].

Maternal undernutrition and inadequate macronutrient intake early in life have been linked to permanent changes in gene expression patterns and long-term changes in the cardiovascular and metabolic functioning of offspring [22, 23]. Therefore, malnutrition during critical developmental stages has the potential to increase the risk of stroke. These long-term health sequels of poorly fed mothers and babies call for increased investment to fight hunger and malnutrition.

Table 6.2. Sustainable Development Goal 2 targets.

2.1
By 2030, end hunger and ensure access by all people, in particular the poor and people in vulnerable situations, including infants, to safe, nutritious and sufficient food all year round.
2.2
By 2030, end all forms of malnutrition, including achieving, by 2025, the internationally agreed targets on stunting and wasting in children under 5 years of age, and address the nutritional needs of adolescent girls, pregnant and lactating women and older persons.
2.3
By 2030, double the agricultural productivity and incomes of small-scale food producers, in particular women, indigenous peoples, family farmers, pastoralists and fishers, including through secure and equal access to land, other productive resources and inputs, knowledge, financial services, markets and opportunities for value addition and non-farm employment.
2.4
By 2030, ensure sustainable food production systems and implement resilient agricultural practices that increase productivity and production, that help maintain ecosystems, that strengthen capacity for adaptation to climate change, extreme weather, drought, flooding and other disasters and that progressively improve land and soil quality.
2.5
By 2020, maintain the genetic diversity of seeds, cultivated plants and farmed and domesticated animals and their related wild species, including through soundly managed and diversified seed and plant banks at the national, regional and international levels, and promote access to and fair and equitable sharing of benefits arising from the utilization of genetic resources and associated traditional knowledge, as internationally agreed.
2.a
Increase investment, including through enhanced international cooperation, in rural infrastructure, agricultural research and extension services, technology development and plant and livestock gene banks in order to enhance agricultural productive capacity in developing countries, in particular least-developed countries.
2.b
Correct and prevent trade restrictions and distortions in world agricultural markets, including through the parallel elimination of all forms of agricultural export subsidies and all export measures with equivalent effect, in accordance with the mandate of the Doha Development Round.
2.c
Adopt measures to ensure the proper functioning of food commodity markets and their derivatives and facilitate timely access to market information, including on food reserves, in order to help limit extreme food price volatility.

Source: United Nations. Sustainable Development Goals Knowledge Platform. https://sustainabledevelopment.un.org

Targets for Goal 2 call countries to adopt measures to increase agricultural productivity, incomes of small-scale food producers and investment in rural agricultural infrastructure and to ensure sustainable food production systems, maintain genetic diversity of plant and animal species, correct trade restrictions in world agricultural markets and facilitate timely access to market information in order to help limit extreme food price volatility.

4.3. Sustainable Development Goal 3

Sustainable Development Goal 3 seeks to ensure health and well-being for all, at every stage of life. As shown in Table **6.3**, Goal 3 addresses all major health priorities, NCDs (stroke); tobacco use, harmful use of alcohol and air pollution; mental health; reproductive, maternal and child health; communicable and environmental diseases; road traffic accidents; and access for all to safe, effective, quality and affordable medicines and vaccines. It also calls for universal health coverage, more research and development and strengthened capacity of all countries in health risk reduction and management. Actions to address these major health priorities are integral to the successful implementation of other Sustainable Development Goals.

According to United Nations data [10, 11] between 2000 and 2015, the number of maternal deaths per 100 000 live births declined by 37%. Although child (under 5) mortality rates declined by 44% globally, an estimated 5.9 million children under 5 died in 2015. Worldwide in 2015, approximately three in four women of reproductive age used modern contraceptive methods. The incidence of major infectious diseases, including HIV, tuberculosis and malaria, has declined globally over the last two decades. Globally, premature mortality from cardiovascular disease, cancer, diabetes and chronic respiratory disease also declined by 15% between 2000 and 2012 [18].

The global prevalence of tobacco smoking among people aged 15 or older is estimated to have declined from 27% in 2000 to 21% in 2013. Declines were largest for men in the Organisation for Economic Co-operation and Development (OECD) high-income countries, and in low-, middle- and non-OECD high-income countries in the WHO Region of the Americas and European Region (all with declines of around 10%) [24]. Going forward, reducing tobacco use through the implementation of the WHO Framework Convention on Tobacco Control will be critical for meeting the proposed target of reducing premature mortality from NCDs by one third by 2030. This framework, ratified in 2005 by 180 Parties, is the first global public health treaty negotiated under the auspices of WHO. It requires its Parties to implement policies and interventions designed to reduce both demand and supply of tobacco products. They include among others: (i) raising taxes on tobacco; (ii) banning smoking in public places; (iii) pictorial health warnings; (iv) banning tobacco advertising; (v) controlling illicit trade of tobacco products; (vi) identifying crops to replace tobacco farming and preventing sales to and by minors; and (vii) collecting and disseminating data on tobacco use and prevention efforts.

One of the targets of Goal 3 is to reduce harmful use of alcohol, which is an important risk factor of stroke. Worldwide, average alcohol consumption in 2015 was estimated at 6.3 litres of pure alcohol per person among those aged 15 or older, with wide variations across countries [18]. Another target of Goal 3, which is closely related to stroke, aims to reduce deaths and illnesses related to air, water and soil pollution and hazardous chemicals. Exposure to indoor (household, due to burning of solid fuels) and outdoor air pollution is a major risk factor for stroke and other NCDs [25]. Worldwide, 3.7 million premature deaths were attributable to outdoor pollution in 2012. Majority of these deaths (about 88%) occurred in developing countries. Between 1980 and 2012, there was a significant reduction in the proportion of households primarily relying on solid fuels for cooking [25]. However, the absolute number of people who use solid fuel primarily for cooking has remained relatively constant over the last three decades at around 3 billion people.

Over the last decade there has been hardly any improvement in outdoor air quality. In 2012, about three quarters of the global population was exposed to particulate matter in concentrations exceeding the WHO Air Quality Guidelines [26, 27]. In many high-income countries, including in Europe and North America, air pollution has declined over the past decades due to efforts to reduce smog-forming emissions and particulate matter. There have been significant declines in air quality in South and East Asia, owing to population growth and increasing industrialization [28].

In May 2015, the World Health Assembly resolution "Addressing the health impacts of air pollution", adopted unanimously by the 194 Member States, aimed to further strengthen efforts and international cooperation to address air pollution and identified key strategic priorities for the future including: (i) developing new energy efficient and affordable technologies such as induction stoves that can reduce household air pollution and related health risks; (ii) strengthening health sector capacity to contribute to multisectoral policy-making that benefits health and air quality; and (iii) improving the monitoring of air quality and identification of pollution sources, including through satellite remote sensing, portable monitors, data mining and crowd sourcing. The Sustainable Development Goals, with air quality dimensions in at least four other goals (Goal 7 on sustainable energy, Goal 9 on sustainable industrialization, Goal 11 on sustainable cities and human settlements and Goal 13 on combating climate change), provide a good platform for integrated efforts to address air pollution and other environmental determinants of NCDs.

The transition to universal health coverage, which is one of the targets of Goal 3, is central to making progress in prevention and control of stroke. Universal health coverage ensures that people can access the health services they need without facing financial hardship. Countries working towards universal health coverage need to build health systems with a strong primary health care base that deliver the quality services and products people need, when and where they need them, through an adequately resourced and competent health workforce. Universal health coverage provides an overall framework for the integration of NCD prevention and treatment services with other health services, including person-centred primary care integrating the WHO Package of Essential NCD Interventions (WHO PEN) interventions [29, 30]. This includes achieving the two NCD health coverage targets of: (i) at least 50% of eligible people receive drug therapy and counselling to prevent heart attacks and strokes; and (ii) at least 80% availability of essential medicines required to treat major NCDs [31]. In addition to the two health coverage targets, the Global NCD Action Plan 2013–2020 has seven other targets [31]. Three targets focus on NCD mortality, tobacco and alcohol, which are also target areas under Sustainable Development Goal 3.

One of the targets of Goal 3 is to substantially increase health financing by 2030 so that as more resources become available, countries can ensure progressive expansion of coverage of health services and financial protection, beyond a minimum package of health services. NCDs (stroke), receive the smallest amount of official development assistance (ODA) among all major global health areas, accounting for 1% of this aid. According to a recent WHO/World Bank Group report, 400 million people do not have access to essential health services and 6% of people in developing countries are tipped into or pushed further into extreme poverty because of health spending [32]. In this regard, the 3rd United Nations International Conference on Financing for Development, held on 13–16 July in Addis Ababa, Ethiopia, resulted in the adoption of an Action Agenda to finance the Sustainable Development Goals. The Addis Ababa Action Agenda presents a policy framework to realign financial flows with public goals [33]. The Action Agenda reiterates the principle that countries have the primary responsibility for investing to attain the Sustainable Development Goals, while the international community has an obligation to create an enabling environment, including through catalytic official development assistance.

Table 6.3. Sustainable Development Goal 3 targets.

3.1 By 2030, reduce the global maternal mortality ratio to less than 70 per 100 000 live births.
3.2 By 2030, end preventable deaths of newborns and children under 5 years of age, with all countries aiming to reduce neonatal mortality to at least as low as 12 per 1000 live births and under-5 mortality to at least as low as 25 per 1000 live births.
3.3 By 2030, end the epidemics of AIDS, tuberculosis, malaria and neglected tropical diseases and combat hepatitis, waterborne diseases and other communicable diseases.
3.4 By 2030, reduce by one third premature mortality from noncommunicable diseases through prevention and treatment and promote mental health and well-being.
3.5 Strengthen the prevention and treatment of substance abuse, including narcotic drug abuse and harmful use of alcohol.
3.6 By 2020, halve the number of global deaths and injuries from road traffic accidents.
3.7 By 2030, ensure universal access to sexual and reproductive health-care services, including for family planning, information and education, and the integration of reproductive health into national strategies and programmes.
3.8 Achieve universal health coverage, including financial risk protection, access to quality essential health-care services and access to safe, effective, quality and affordable essential medicines and vaccines for all.
3.9 By 2030, substantially reduce the number of deaths and illnesses from hazardous chemicals and air, water and soil pollution and contamination.
3.a Strengthen the implementation of the World Health Organization Framework Convention on Tobacco Control in all countries, as appropriate.
3.b Support the research and development of vaccines and medicines for the communicable and noncommunicable diseases that primarily affect developing countries, provide access to affordable essential medicines and vaccines, in accordance with the Doha Declaration on the TRIPS Agreement and Public Health, which affirms the right of developing countries to use to the full the provisions in the Agreement on Trade-Related Aspects of Intellectual Property Rights regarding flexibilities to protect public health, and, in particular, provide access to medicines for all.
3.c Substantially increase health financing and the recruitment, development, training and retention of the health workforce in developing countries, especially in least-developed countries and small island developing States.
3.d Strengthen the capacity of all countries, in particular developing countries, for early warning, risk reduction and management of national and global health risks.

Source: United Nations. Sustainable Development Goals Knowledge Platform.
https://sustainabledevelopment.un.org

4.4. Sustainable Development Goal 4

Sustainable Development Goal 4 aims to ensure inclusive and quality education for all and promote lifelong learning (Table **6.4**). Investing in education results in significant health and development benefits. Education improves access to opportunities. It increases a person's chance of leading an economically gainful, healthy and productive life. It has been proven to reduce maternal mortality and alleviate poverty [34]. Substantial progress has been made towards increasing access to education and enrolment rates in schools. According to United Nations data, the total enrolment rate in low- and middle-income countries reached 91% in 2015, and the number of children out of school had dropped by almost 50%. However, 59 million children of primary school age were out of school in 2013. Completion rates for primary education exceeded 90% in 2013 [34]. Out-o--school rates are also higher among children from poorer households. Progress has been inadequate in some low-income countries due to high levels of poverty, ongoing armed conflicts and disasters. At the end of primary school, children should be able to read and write and do basic mathematics. However, in 2014, between 40% and 90% of children failed to achieve even minimum levels of proficiency in reading and mathematics in 9 African countries [34]. Worldwide, in 2013, two thirds of the 757 million adults who were illiterate were women.

Goal 4 aims to support education so that by 2030 all girls and boys complete free primary and secondary schooling. It also aims to eliminate gender and income disparities, and achieve universal access to a quality higher education.

Education enhances health literacy by improving people's ability to understand and follow health information and to avoid health-harming behaviours. Further, because education can reach children at a young age, it has the potential to catalyse the adoption of healthy behaviours. Attainment of this goal therefore impacts on prevention and control of stroke and other NCDs. One of the targets of Goal 4 is to ensure that all youth and a substantial proportion of both men and women achieve literacy and numeracy. Health literacy enables people to navigate the health-care system, communicate with health-care providers and engage in self-care for NCDs (stroke). Improving health literacy in populations provides the foundation on which people are empowered to play an active participatory role to improve their own health. Higher levels of health literacy within populations is necessary to mobilize society to hold governments accountable to meet their responsibilities in addressing health, including NCDs.

Table 6.4. Sustainable Development Goal 4 targets.

4.1 By 2030, ensure that all girls and boys complete free, equitable and quality primary and secondary education leading to relevant and effective learning outcomes. **4.2** By 2030, ensure that all girls and boys have access to quality early childhood development, care and pre-primary education so that they are ready for primary education. **4.3** By 2030, ensure equal access for all women and men to affordable and quality technical, vocational and tertiary education, including university. **4.4** By 2030, substantially increase the number of youth and adults who have relevant skills, including technical and vocational skills, for employment, decent jobs and entrepreneurship. **4.5** By 2030, eliminate gender disparities in education and ensure equal access to all levels of education and vocational training for the vulnerable, including persons with disabilities, indigenous peoples and children in vulnerable situations. **4.6** By 2030, ensure that all youth and a substantial proportion of adults, both men and women, achieve literacy and numeracy. **4.7** By 2030, ensure that all learners acquire the knowledge and skills needed to promote sustainable development, including, among others, through education for sustainable development and sustainable lifestyles, human rights, gender equality, promotion of a culture of peace and non-violence, global citizenship and appreciation of cultural diversity and of culture's contribution to sustainable development. **4.a** Build and upgrade education facilities that are child, disability and gender sensitive and provide safe, non-violent, inclusive and effective learning environments for all. **4.b** By 2020, substantially expand globally the number of scholarships available to developing countries, in particular least-developed countries, small island developing States and African countries, for enrolment in higher education, including vocational training and information and communications technology, technical, engineering and scientific programmes, in developed countries and other developing countries. **4.c** By 2030, substantially increase the supply of qualified teachers, including through international cooperation for teacher training in developing countries, especially least-developed countries and small island developing States.

Source: United Nations. Sustainable Development Goals Knowledge Platform.
https://sustainabledevelopment.un.org

4.5. Sustainable Development Goal 5

Sustainable Development Goal 5 aims to achieve gender equality and empower all women and girls (Table **6.5**). Gender inequality remains a major barrier to sustainable development. While both men and women face disparities, worldwide, women experience a majority of disparities. In many cultures women have fewer opportunities than men in education, employment and participation in politics. Worldwide, women contribute more than men to unpaid work, including caregiving and domestic work. On average, women report that they spend 19% of their time each day in unpaid activities, *versus* 8% for men [34, 35]. The responsibilities of unpaid caregiving and household chores, often combined with paid employment, means less time for rest, self-care, personal development and social activities. Violence against women and girls violates their human rights and hinders development. According to WHO estimates, about one in three (35%) women worldwide have experienced either physical and/or sexual intimate partner violence or non-partner sexual violence in their lifetime. Additionally, human trafficking disproportionately affects women and girls, since 70% of all victims detected worldwide are female [36].

In recent years, improvements have been reported in girls' access to education, the rate of child marriage, sexual and reproductive health and reproductive rights and maternal mortality. The rate of marriage of girls under age 15 has declined globally from 12% around 1990 to 7% around 2015 [37]. Ensuring women's rights through legal frameworks is a key step in tackling discrimination against them. As of 2014, 143 countries guaranteed equality between men and women in their constitutions; another 52 countries have yet to make this important commitment [38].

This goal is particularly significant in relation to stroke because a growing body of evidence reveal gender disparities in stroke. There is a significantly higher rate of stroke in older women than in their age-matched male counterparts [39 - 41]. Lower socioeconomic status and poorer living conditions of females account for part of these sex disparities in stroke [38, 39, 42 - 44].

Elderly women, compared to men, have a longer pre-hospital stay and are less likely to be admitted to the acute stroke care unit within the eligible time that may potentially delay treatment and result in poor stroke outcomes [38, 39, 45 - 47].

Elderly women are not evaluated the same as elderly men are and possibly not treated appropriately. Women were less likely to have echocardiography or any carotid investigation. They were also less likely to be treated with antithrombotic drugs and less likely to receive anticoagulation [48, 49]. The in-hospital stroke mortality rate among elderly women is at least three times higher than that among men [45, 50].

Women also have significantly worse functional outcomes after stroke compared to men [51]. The most important factor attenuating the difference is functional status before the stroke. Prevention efforts aimed at maintaining pre-stroke functional status in elderly women could improve their stroke outcomes. The determinants of these disparities include low income status and health literacy, poor access to health insurance and pre-stroke functional status, and lack of gender sensitivity of clinicians. Efforts focused in attaining Goal 5 will indirectly contribute to eliminating the root causes of these gender disparities in stroke.

Table 6.5. Sustainable Development Goal 5 targets.

5.1 End all forms of discrimination against all women and girls everywhere.
5.2 Eliminate all forms of violence against all women and girls in the public and private spheres, including trafficking and sexual and other types of exploitation.
5.3 Eliminate all harmful practices, such as child, early and forced marriage and female genital mutilation.
5.4 Recognize and value unpaid care and domestic work through the provision of public services, infrastructure and social protection policies and the promotion of shared responsibility within the household and the family as nationally appropriate.
5.5 Ensure women's full and effective participation and equal opportunities for leadership at all levels of decision-making in political, economic and public life.
5.6 Ensure universal access to sexual and reproductive health and reproductive rights as agreed in accordance with the Programme of Action of the International Conference on Population and Development and the Beijing Platform for Action and the outcome documents of their review conferences.
5.a Undertake reforms to give women equal rights to economic resources, as well as access to ownership and control over land and other forms of property, financial services, inheritance and natural resources, in accordance with national laws.
5.b Enhance the use of enabling technology, in particular information and communications technology, to promote the empowerment of women.
5.c Adopt and strengthen sound policies and enforceable legislation for the promotion of gender equality and the empowerment of all women and girls at all levels.

Source: United Nations. Sustainable Development Goals Knowledge Platform. https://sustainabledevelopment.un.org

4.6. Sustainable Development Goal 6

Sustainable Development Goal 6 is to ensure availability and sustainable management of water and sanitation for all (Table **6.6**). Water and sanitation are critical to the existence of people and are at the heart of sustainable development. Goal 6 addresses the issues relating to drinking water, sanitation and hygiene, as well as ensures the sustainability of water resources worldwide. The unsafe management of faecal waste and wastewater continues to be a major public health and environment issue. In 2015, 946 million people did not have any sanitation facilities and continued to practise open defecation [10, 11].

Less than 0.01% of all water worldwide is available for human use in lakes, rivers and reservoirs [11]. The total annual average requirement of water per person has been estimated at 1000 cubic metres [52]. In 1990, 11 countries in Africa and the Middle East had less than 1000 cubic metres of freshwater available per person [11, 52]. Inadequate access to safe drinking water contributes to communicable disease, kidney disease and even stroke [53]. Many countries are dependent on water resources that originate from outside their national territory, which can be a potential source for intercountry conflicts [54].

Table 6.6. Sustainable Development Goal 6 targets.

6.1
By 2030, achieve universal and equitable access to safe and affordable drinking water for all.
6.2
By 2030, achieve access to adequate and equitable sanitation and hygiene for all and end open defecation, paying special attention to the needs of women and girls and those in vulnerable situations.
6.3
By 2030, improve water quality by reducing pollution, eliminating dumping and minimizing release of hazardous chemicals and materials, halving the proportion of untreated wastewater and substantially increasing recycling and safe reuse globally.
6.4
By 2030, substantially increase water-use efficiency across all sectors and ensure sustainable withdrawals and supply of freshwater to address water scarcity and substantially reduce the number of people suffering from water scarcity.
6.5
By 2030, implement integrated water resources management at all levels, including through transboundary cooperation as appropriate.
6.6
By 2020, protect and restore water-related ecosystems, including mountains, forests, wetlands, rivers, aquifers and lakes.
6.a
By 2030, expand international cooperation and capacity-building support to developing countries in water- and sanitation-related activities and programmes, including water harvesting, desalination, water efficiency, wastewater treatment, recycling and reuse technologies.
6.b
Support and strengthen the participation of local communities in improving water and sanitation management.

Source: United Nations. Sustainable Development Goals Knowledge Platform. https://sustainabledevelopment.un.org

According to United Nations data, improvements have been made in access to drinking water. In 2015, 6.6 billion people, or 91% of the global population, used an improved drinking water source, but not all improved sources are safe [10, 11]. For example, in 2012 it was estimated that at least 1.8 billion people were exposed to drinking water sources contaminated with faecal matter.

Public health workers can play significant roles in ensuring equitable access to freshwater [55, 56]. These roles include: (i) raising awareness about the importance of access to freshwater and its efficient use; (ii) promoting non-violent ways to resolving disagreements over water; (iii) strengthening efforts to prevent contamination of water; (iv) promoting proactive cooperation among countries; and (v) supporting the attainment of Sustainable Development Goal 6.

4.7. Sustainable Development Goal 7

Sustainable Development Goal 7 is to ensure access to affordable, reliable, sustainable and modern energy for all (Table **6.7**). Energy is critical for achieving most of the other Sustainable Development Goals. Access to electricity is essential for implementing most of the technological advances in medicine, including for the treatment of acute stroke and stroke rehabilitation.

Table 6.7. Sustainable Development Goal 7 targets.

7.1 By 2030, ensure universal access to affordable, reliable and modern energy services.
7.2 By 2030, increase substantially the share of renewable energy in the global energy mix.
7.3 By 2030, double the global rate of improvement in energy efficiency.
7.a By 2030, enhance international cooperation to facilitate access to clean energy research and technology, including renewable energy, energy efficiency and advanced and cleaner fossil-fuel technology, and promote investment in energy infrastructure and clean energy technology.
7.b By 2030, expand infrastructure and upgrade technology for supplying modern and sustainable energy services for all in developing countries, in particular least-developed countries, small island developing States, and land-locked developing countries, in accordance with their respective programmes of support.

Source: United Nations. Sustainable Development Goals Knowledge Platform.
https://sustainabledevelopment.un.org

According to United Nations data, globally one in five people still lacks access to electricity. At least 3 billion people rely on solid fuels such as wood, coal, charcoal or animal waste for domestic needs. Energy is the main contributor to climate change, accounting for around 60% of total global greenhouse gas emissions [10, 11]. The proportion of the world's population with access to electricity has risen from 79% in 2000 to 85% in 2012 [10, 11, 57]. The proportion of the global population with access to clean fuels increased to 58% in 2014 [11, 57]. The share of renewable energy (derived from hydropower, wind, sun, biofuels, biogas and geothermal sources, and waste) in the world's total final energy consumption has increased in recent years. Hydropower, wind and solar power together accounted for 73% of the total increase in modern renewable energy between 2010 and 2012 [57].

4.8. Sustainable Development Goal 8

Sustainable Development Goal 8 aims to promote inclusive and sustainable economic growth and employment (Table **6.8**). Continued inclusive economic growth is necessary for achieving sustainable development. Economic development, employment and access to financial services are essential components of inclusive growth. The global annual growth rate of real GDP per person increased by 1.3% in 2014 [10, 11]. Sustainable economic growth necessitates the creation of job opportunities across the whole working-age population to boost the economy, while protecting the environment. Economic growth, employment and health are closely linked because national income and labour markets have direct effects on the financing and performance of health systems, through insurance coverage and public spending on health. Stroke and other NCDs affect economic growth through three main channels [58]. First, NCDs can increase health expenditures for households, companies and governments. Second, NCDs exert a negative macroeconomic impact through labour and productivity losses. Third, NCDs affect the incentives for savings and for investment in both physical and human capital [58].

In 2015, the global unemployment rate was 6.1%. Worldwide, unemployment affects women and youth are more than men and adults aged 25 or over. Labour productivity hastens economic growth. Despite rapid growth in some developing regions, labour productivity remains far higher in developed regions. In 2015, the average worker in developed regions produced 23 times the annual output of an average worker in developing regions such as sub-Saharan Africa.

Between 2011 and 2014, 700 million adults became account holders, increasing the proportion of the world's adult population with an account at a financial institution or a mobile money service provider from 51% to 62% [11].

4.9. Sustainable Development Goal 9

Sustainable Development Goal 9 aims to build resilient infrastructure and promote sustainable industrialization (Table **6.9**). This goal incorporates three key drivers of economic growth and sustainable development: infrastructure; industrialization; and innovation. Infrastructure provides the basic physical systems and structures essential to the operation of a society or business. Lack of infrastructure is a barrier to productivity as it reduces access to jobs, markets, training, education and health care and thus creating a barrier to doing business. Industrialization drives economic growth, creates employment and thereby reduces income poverty. Innovation advances the technological capabilities of industrial sectors and promotes the growth of new industries.

Table 6.8. Sustainable Development Goal 8 targets.

8.1
Sustain per capita economic growth in accordance with national circumstances and, in particular, at least 7 per cent gross domestic product growth per annum in the least-developed countries.
8.2
Achieve higher levels of economic productivity through diversification, technological upgrading and innovation, including through a focus on high-value added and labour-intensive sectors.
8.3
Promote development-oriented policies that support productive activities, decent job creation, entrepreneurship, creativity and innovation, and encourage the formalization and growth of micro-, small- and medium-sized enterprises, including through access to financial services.
8.4
Improve progressively, through 2030, global resource efficiency in consumption and production and endeavour to decouple economic growth from environmental degradation, in accordance with the 10-year framework of programmes on sustainable consumption and production, with developed countries taking the lead.
8.5
By 2030, achieve full and productive employment and decent work for all women and men, including for young people and persons with disabilities, and equal pay for work of equal value.
8.6
By 2020, substantially reduce the proportion of youth not in employment, education or training.
8.7
Take immediate and effective measures to eradicate forced labour, end modern slavery and human trafficking and secure the prohibition and elimination of the worst forms of child labour, including recruitment and use of child soldiers, and by 2025 end child labour in all its forms.
8.8
Protect labour rights and promote safe and secure working environments for all workers, including migrant workers, in particular women migrants, and those in precarious employment.
8.9
By 2030, devise and implement policies to promote sustainable tourism that creates jobs and promotes local culture and products.
8.10
Strengthen the capacity of domestic financial institutions to encourage and expand access to banking, insurance and financial services for all.
8.a
Increase Aid for Trade support for developing countries, in particular least-developed countries, including through the Enhanced Integrated Framework for Trade-Related Technical Assistance to Least Developed Countries.
8.b
By 2020, develop and operationalize a global strategy for youth employment and implement the Global Jobs Pact of the International Labour Organization.

Source: United Nations. Sustainable Development Goals Knowledge Platform. https://sustainabledevelopment.un.org

Table 6.9. Sustainable Development Goal 9.

9.1 Develop quality, reliable, sustainable and resilient infrastructure, including regional and transborder infrastructure, to support economic development and human well-being, with a focus on affordable and equitable access for all.
9.2 Promote inclusive and sustainable industrialization and, by 2030, significantly raise industry's share of employment and gross domestic product, in line with national circumstances, and double its share in least-developed countries.
9.3 Increase the access of small-scale industrial and other enterprises, in particular in developing countries, to financial services, including affordable credit, and their integration into value chains and markets.
9.4 By 2030, upgrade infrastructure and retrofit industries to make them sustainable, with increased resource-use efficiency and greater adoption of clean and environmentally sound technologies and industrial processes, with all countries taking action in accordance with their respective capabilities.
9.5 Enhance scientific research, upgrade the technological capabilities of industrial sectors in all countries, in particular developing countries, including, by 2030, encouraging innovation and substantially increasing the number of research and development workers per 1 million people and public and private research and development spending.
9.a Facilitate sustainable and resilient infrastructure development in developing countries through enhanced financial, technological and technical support to African countries, least-developed countries, landlocked developing countries and small island developing States.
9.b Support domestic technology development, research and innovation in developing countries, including by ensuring a conducive policy environment for, inter alia, industrial diversification and value addition to commodities.
9.c Significantly increase access to information and communications technology and strive to provide universal and affordable access to the Internet in least-developed countries by 2020.

Source: United Nations. Sustainable Development Goals Knowledge Platform.
https://sustainabledevelopment.un.org

Progress of information and communication technologies (ICT) are important for finding pragmatic solutions to economic challenges, such as providing new jobs. Progress of information and communication technologies can impact positively on the environment by promoting energy efficiency. On the other hand there are also environmental challenges related to the fallout from the processes of production of information and communication technologies, and the environmental burden of the ICT products themselves and their use. Promoting sustainable industries, and investing in scientific research and innovation, are all important and promising ways to facilitate sustainable development.

Information and communication can help to empower the masses through knowledge dissemination and transform the world. The internet is a powerful vehicle which can jump-start this process. However, more than 4 billion people still do not have access to the Internet, and 90% are from the developing world. Decreasing the cost and increasing the ease of internet use can bridge this digital divide to ensure equal access to information and knowledge and also foster innovation and entrepreneurship [1]. One of the targets of Goal 9 is to increase by significant rates access to information and communication technology, and work towards providing affordable universal access to the Internet in developing countries, especially the least-developed ones by 2020.

Innovation and the creation of new and more sustainable industries require investments in research and development. In 2012, expenditure on research and development was 2.4% of GDP for developed regions, 1.2% for developing regions and below 0.3% for the least-developed countries [11]. The number of researchers per 1 million inhabitants ranged from 65 per 1 million in the least-developed countries to 3641 per 1 million in developed regions.

Increasing investment in infrastructure and innovation is also critical for prevention and control of NCDs, (stroke). Multisectoral action required for addressing NCDs cannot succeed without investment in resilient infrastructure, institutional support, and research and development, which are specific targets of Goal 9. Weak capacity for research and development is a major impediment for NCD prevention and control. Although effective interventions exist for the prevention and control of NCDs, application of these interventions worldwide has to be supported by context-specific research.

4.10. Sustainable Development Goal 10

Sustainable Development Goal 10 aims to reduce inequality within and among countries (Table **6.10**). This goal calls for reducing inequalities in income as well as those based on age, sex, disability, race, ethnicity, origin, religion or economic status within a country. It also addresses inequalities among countries, including those related to representation, migration and development assistance.

According to United Nations data, inequality is on the rise, with the richest 10% earning up to 40% of total global income. The poorest 10% earn only between 2% and 7% of total global income [11]. Evidence from developing countries shows that children in the poorest 20% of the populations have a three-fold risk of dying before their fifth birthday than children in the richest quintiles.

New research shows that when **income inequality** rises, **economic growth** falls and that inequality is detrimental to poverty reduction. To tackle income inequality, the underlying inequality of opportunities needs to be addressed through the adoption of wide-ranging policies to empower the bottom percentile of income earners and promote economic inclusion of all regardless of sex, race or ethnicity. Anti-poverty programmes and better access to public services, such as quality education, housing and healthcare, are essential to create greater equality of opportunities for the poorest 10 per cent of the population.

Table 6.10. Sustainable Development Goal 10 targets.

10.1
By 2030, progressively achieve and sustain income growth of the bottom 40 per cent of the population at a rate higher than the national average.
10.2
By 2030, empower and promote the social, economic and political inclusion of all, irrespective of age, sex, disability, race, ethnicity, origin, religion or economic or other status.
10.3
Ensure equal opportunity and reduce inequalities of outcome, including by eliminating discriminatory laws, policies and practices and promoting appropriate legislation, policies and action in this regard.
10.4
Adopt policies, especially fiscal, wage and social protection policies, and progressively achieve greater equality.
10.5
Improve the regulation and monitoring of global financial markets and institutions and strengthen the implementation of such regulations.
10.6
Ensure enhanced representation and voice for developing countries in decision-making in global international economic and financial institutions in order to deliver more effective, credible, accountable and legitimate institutions.
10.7
Facilitate orderly, safe, regular and responsible migration and mobility of people, including through the implementation of planned and well-managed migration policies.
10.a
Implement the principle of special and differential treatment for developing countries, in particular least-developed countries, in accordance with World Trade Organization agreements.
10.b
Encourage official development assistance and financial flows, including foreign direct investment, to States where the need is greatest, in particular least-developed countries, African countries, small island developing States and landlocked developing countries, in accordance with their national plans and programmes.
10.c
By 2030, reduce to less than 3 percent the transaction costs of migrant remittances and eliminate remittance corridors with costs higher than 5 percent.

Source: United Nations. Sustainable Development Goals Knowledge Platform.
https://sustainabledevelopment.un.org

One of the targets of Goal 10 seeks to ensure that income growth among the poorest 40% of the population in every country is more rapid than its national average [11]. This involves improving the regulation and monitoring of financial markets and institutions, encouraging development assistance and foreign direct investment to the poorest regions of the world.

Official development assistance contributes to reducing inequalities within and among countries. In 2014, total resource flows for development to the least-developed countries totalled US$ 55.2 billion, and eight donor countries met the target of 0.15% of gross national income (GNI) for official development assistance to the least-developed countries [11].

Advances in prevention and control have driven the decline in morbidity and mortality from cardiovascular disease, including stroke, since the 1970s [18]. However, these benefits have not been spread evenly across populations owing to inequalities within and between countries. Rates of illness and premature death are significantly higher among the poorest and most marginalized groups. Efforts in attaining Goal 10 will help to alleviate inequalities within and among countries that are barriers to prevention and treatment of stroke through better access to education, income and health care.

4.11. Sustainable Development Goal 11

Sustainable Development Goal 11 aims to make cities and human settlements inclusive, safe, resilient and sustainable (Table **6.11**). By 2030, it is projected that 6 out of 10 people will live in cities. As more people migrate to cities in search of employment and urban populations grow, cities expand beyond the formal administrative boundaries and demands and needs of city dwellers intensify [11]. In 2014, 30% of the urban population lived in slum-like conditions and globally more than 880 million people were living in slums in 2014.

WHO has identified urbanization as one of the key challenges for public health in the 21st century [59]. Decisions related to urban planning and governance can increase the exposure of populations to major health risks – or they can promote healthier environments and lifestyles that in turn prevent both communicable diseases and NCDs [59]. Urban policies that lead to increased air pollution contribute to premature deaths from strokes, and other NCDs. In 2014, around half the global urban population was exposed to air pollution levels at least 2.5 times higher than maximum standards set by WHO [11]. Only 12% of cities globally reach pollution control targets [59]. Poorly managed waste and stagnant water worsen the transmission of communicable diseases. Outmoded transport strategies contribute to air pollution and road traffic accidents. On the other hand, urban planning that protects health – for example, by improving the physical environment, access to safe, green spaces, and controlling the sources of pollution – offers significant opportunities for improving the economic productivity, physical activity levels and health of urban populations [60 - 62]. Health-promoting urban policies also reduce social inequalities through better access to housing, employment, jobs, safe transport, and education [59 - 62]. The WHO

Healthy Cities programme has become an important platform for achieving health and sustainable development in many parts of the world, with mayors and municipalities leading efforts to improve the daily living conditions of city dwellers [59]. To attain the targets covered under this goal national development planning have to focus on improving housing, transport systems, cities and public spaces, resilience to disasters and protecting cultural and natural heritage.

Table 11. Sustainable Development Goal 11 targets.

11.1 By 2030, ensure access for all to adequate, safe and affordable housing and basic services and upgrade slums.
11.2 By 2030, provide access to safe, affordable, accessible and sustainable transport systems for all, improving road safety, notably by expanding public transport, with special attention to the needs of those in vulnerable situations, women, children, persons with disabilities and older persons.
11.3 By 2030, enhance inclusive and sustainable urbanization and capacity for participatory, integrated and sustainable human settlement planning and management in all countries.
11.4 Strengthen efforts to protect and safeguard the world's cultural and natural heritage.
11.5 By 2030, significantly reduce the number of deaths and the number of people affected and substantially decrease the direct economic losses relative to global gross domestic product caused by disasters, including water-related disasters, with a focus on protecting the poor and people in vulnerable situations.
11.6 By 2030, reduce the adverse per capita environmental impact of cities, including by paying special attention to air quality and municipal and other waste management.
11.7 By 2030, provide universal access to safe, inclusive and accessible, green and public spaces, in particular for women and children, older persons and persons with disabilities.
11.a Support positive economic, social and environmental links between urban, peri-urban and rural areas by strengthening national and regional development planning.
11.b By 2020, substantially increase the number of cities and human settlements adopting and implementing integrated policies and plans towards inclusion, resource efficiency, mitigation and adaptation to climate change, resilience to disasters, and develop and implement, in line with the Sendai Framework for Disaster Risk Reduction 2015–2030, holistic disaster risk management at all levels.
11.c Support least-developed countries, including through financial and technical assistance, in building sustainable and resilient buildings utilizing local materials.

Source: United Nations. Sustainable Development Goals Knowledge Platform.
https://sustainabledevelopment.un.org

4.12. Sustainable Development Goal 12

Sustainable Development Goal 12 is to ensure sustainable consumption and production patterns (Table **6.12**). Achieving economic growth and sustainable development requires that we reduce our ecological footprint by managing the way goods and resources are produced and consumed. Reckless consumption and production patterns have a negative impact on the climate, the environment, and on the health of populations.

Table 6.12. Sustainable Development Goal 12 targets.

12.1
Implement the 10-year framework of programmes on sustainable consumption and production, all countries taking action, with developed countries taking the lead, taking into account the development and capabilities of developing countries.
12.2
By 2030, achieve the sustainable management and efficient use of natural resources.
12.3
By 2030, halve per capita global food waste at the retail and consumer levels and reduce food losses along production and supply chains, including post-harvest losses.
12.4
By 2020, achieve the environmentally sound management of chemicals and all wastes throughout their life cycle, in accordance with agreed international frameworks, and significantly reduce their release to air, water and soil in order to minimize their adverse impacts on human health and the environment.
12.5
By 2030, substantially reduce waste generation through prevention, reduction, recycling and reuse.
12.6
Encourage companies, especially large and transnational companies, to adopt sustainable practices and to integrate sustainability information into their reporting cycle.
12.7
Promote public procurement practices that are sustainable, in accordance with national policies and priorities.
12.8
By 2030, ensure that people everywhere have the relevant information and awareness for sustainable development and lifestyles in harmony with nature.
12.a
Support developing countries to strengthen their scientific and technological capacity to move towards more sustainable patterns of consumption and production.
12.b
Develop and implement tools to monitor sustainable development impacts for sustainable tourism that creates jobs and promotes local culture and products.
12.c
Rationalize inefficient fossil-fuel subsidies that encourage wasteful consumption by removing market distortions, in accordance with national circumstances, including by restructuring taxation and phasing out those harmful subsidies, where they exist, to reflect their environmental impacts, taking fully into account the specific needs and conditions of developing countries and minimizing the possible adverse impacts on their development in a manner that protects the poor and the affected communities.

Source: United Nations. Sustainable Development Goals Knowledge Platform.
https://sustainabledevelopment.un.org

Degradation of land and marine environments, declining soil fertility, unsustainable water use and overfishing are rapidly exhausting the natural resource base of the Earth. Currently, 1.3 billion tonnes of food are lost or wasted every year, while almost 800 million people go hungry [10, 11]. Toxic chemicals, nuclear waste, and degrading pesticides are dumped in various locations in Africa, Asia, Eastern Europe and Latin America and pollute the environment [63].

International frameworks, including the Basel Convention, the Rotterdam Convention and the Stockholm Convention, have been established to achieve the environmentally sound management of hazardous wastes, chemicals and persistent organic pollutants. The Basel Convention on the Control of Transboundary Movements of Hazardous Wastes and their Disposal was adopted on 22 March 1989 [64]. The Stockholm Convention is an international environmental treaty, signed in 2001, that aims to eliminate or restrict the production and use of persistent organic pollutants [65]. The Rotterdam Convention, adopted on 10 September 1998, is a multilateral treaty that assists Parties to reduce risks from certain hazardous pesticides in international trade [66]. There are now 183 Parties to the Basel Convention, 180 to the Stockholm Convention and 155 to the Rotterdam Convention.

The efficient management of natural resources, and safe disposal of toxic waste and pollutants are important targets to achieve Goal 12. Encouraging industries, and consumers to recycle and reduce waste is equally important, as is supporting countries to move towards more sustainable patterns of consumption by 2030.

4.13. Sustainable Development Goal 13

Sustainable Development Goal 13 aims to take urgent action to combat climate change and its impacts (Table **6.13**). The United Nations Framework Convention on Climate Change (UNFCCC) defines "climate change" as "a change of climate which is attributed directly or indirectly to human activity that alters the composition of the global atmosphere and which is in addition to natural climate variability observed over comparable time periods" [67].

The Earth's climate is changing rapidly, resulting in rising temperatures and sea levels, changing patterns of rainfall and frequent and severe weather events. The primary cause of climate change is the burning of fossil fuels, which emits greenhouse gases into the atmosphere. Other human activities, such as agriculture and deforestation, also contribute to the rise in greenhouse gases that cause climate change. Greenhouse gases such as carbon dioxide, methane and water vapour absorb energy, slowing loss of heat from the Earth and making it warmer than it would otherwise be.

Climate change presents a major threat to development. Effects of climate change are widespread and impacts the poorest and most vulnerable disproportionately. Climate change is already affecting the most vulnerable countries and populations, in particular the least-developed countries and the small island developing states. Between 1990 and 2013, more than 1.6 million people died in internationally reported disasters [11].

Table 6.13. Sustainable Development Goal 13 targets.

13.1
Strengthen resilience and adaptive capacity to climate-related hazards and natural disasters in all countries.
13.2
Integrate climate change measures into national policies, strategies and planning
13.3
Improve education, awareness-raising and human and institutional capacity on climate change mitigation, adaptation, impact reduction and early warning.
13.a
Implement the commitment undertaken by developed-country parties to the United Nations Framework Convention on Climate Change* to a goal of mobilizing jointly US$ 100 billion annually by 2020 from all sources to address the needs of developing countries in the context of meaningful mitigation actions and transparency on implementation and fully operationalize the Green Climate Fund through its capitalization as soon as possible.
13.b
Promote mechanisms for raising capacity for effective climate change-related planning and management in least-developed countries and small island developing States, including focusing on women, youth and local and marginalized communities.
* Acknowledging that the United Nations Framework Convention on Climate Change is the primary international, intergovernmental forum for negotiating the global response to climate change.

Source: United Nations. Sustainable Development Goals Knowledge Platform. https://sustainabledevelopment.un.org

Climate change can affect human health through several mechanisms, including relatively direct effects of hazards such as floods and storms, and more complex pathways of altered infectious disease patterns, disruptions of agricultural and other supportive ecosystems, and potentially population displacement and conflict over depleted resources such as water, fertile land and fisheries [68].

On 22 April 2016, 175 Member States signed the Paris Agreement under the United Nations Framework Convention on Climate Change [69]. The new agreement aims to reduce the pace of climate change by actions and investments that develop sustainable low-carbon pathways and accelerate the reduction of global greenhouse gas emissions. Many countries have already taken steps to integrate climate change measures into national policies and planning.

As Parties scale up climate change action, enhanced cooperation, capacity-building and access to financial and technical support will be needed to help less-developed countries to realize their priorities. Developed countries have committed to mobilizing, by 2020, US$ 100 billion per year in climate financing to help address the needs of developing countries.

Climate change and NCDs (stroke), are closely linked and present shared opportunities for joint action in several key areas: energy; air pollution; transport; and food systems [70]. Interventions in these four key areas have beneficial effects on NCDs as well as climate change. As envisioned in Goal 7, increasing the share of renewable energy in the global energy mix is critical for sustainable development. This transition from fossil fuels to renewable energy is also of vital importance for reducing chronic respiratory disease due to indoor air pollution. Air pollution is a leading cause of climate change as well stroke and heart disease. Motorized transport contributes to air pollution. Promoting active transport such as walking and cycling in place of motorized transport has the dual benefit of reducing both air pollution and physical inactivity. Livestock production emits considerable amounts of all three greenhouse gases: carbon dioxide, methane and nitrous oxide. Promoting plant-based diets in place of animal protein-based diets both prevent NCDs and climate change.

4.14. Sustainable Development Goal 14

Sustainable Development Goal 14 aims to conserve and sustainably use the oceans, seas and marine resources for sustainable development (Table **6.14**). Oceans cover three quarters of the surface of the Earth. They are particularly important for social and economic development of people living in coastal areas. Over 3 billion people depend on marine and coastal biodiversity for their livelihoods. Oceans provide their main source of protein. Oceans also absorb heat and one third of the carbon dioxide released by human activities from the atmosphere. This helps to protect coastal areas from flooding and erosion. As much as 40% of the world's oceans are adversely affected by human activities, including pollution, overfishing and loss of coastal habitats [11]. Marine pollution from land-based sources is reaching alarming levels. For example, it is estimated that an average of 13 000 pieces of plastic litters every square kilometre of ocean [71]. Due to pollution, mercury levels in the sea have risen about 30% over the past 20 years [72]. Fish and shellfish concentrate mercury in their bodies that is absorbed into the blood stream when seafood is consumed. High levels consumed over a long period of time accumulate in the body, which can result in mercury poisoning.

Biodiverse marine sites need protection to ensure sustainable long-term use of their natural resources. Globally in 2014, 8.4% of the marine environment was under national control (up to 200 nautical miles from shore) and 0.25% of the marine environment beyond national jurisdiction was under protection [11]. The sustainable use and preservation of marine and coastal ecosystems and their biological diversity are central to achieving the 2030 Agenda for Sustainable Development, in particular for small island developing states.

To attain this goal countries have to make strategic changes in the management of marine and coastal ecosystems to improve conservation and reduce marine pollution and overfishing. The challenge is to balance human needs with conservation.

Table 6.14. Sustainable Development Goal 14 targets.

14.1
By 2025, prevent and significantly reduce marine pollution of all kinds, in particular from land-based activities, including marine debris and nutrient pollution.
14.2
By 2020, sustainably manage and protect marine and coastal ecosystems to avoid significant adverse impacts, including by strengthening their resilience, and take action for their restoration in order to achieve healthy and productive oceans.
14.3
Minimize and address the impacts of ocean acidification, including through enhanced scientific cooperation at all levels.
14.4
By 2020, effectively regulate harvesting and end overfishing, illegal, unreported and unregulated fishing and destructive fishing practices and implement science-based management plans, in order to restore fish stocks in the shortest time feasible, at least to levels that can produce maximum sustainable yield as determined by their biological characteristics.
14.5
By 2020, conserve at least 10 per cent of coastal and marine areas, consistent with national and international law and based on the best available scientific information.
14.6
By 2020, prohibit certain forms of fisheries subsidies which contribute to overcapacity and overfishing, eliminate subsidies that contribute to illegal, unreported and unregulated fishing and refrain from introducing new such subsidies, recognizing that appropriate and effective special and differential treatment for developing and least-developed countries should be an integral part of the World Trade Organization fisheries subsidies negotiation.
14.7
By 2030, increase the economic benefits to Small Island developing States and least-developed countries from the sustainable use of marine resources, including through sustainable management of fisheries, aquaculture and tourism.
14.a
Increase scientific knowledge, develop research capacity and transfer marine technology, taking into account the Intergovernmental Oceanographic Commission Criteria and Guidelines on the Transfer of Marine Technology, in order to improve ocean health and to enhance the contribution of marine biodiversity to the development of developing countries, in particular small island developing States and least-developed countries.
14.b
Provide access for small-scale artisanal fishers to marine resources and markets.
14.c
Enhance the conservation and sustainable use of oceans and their resources by implementing international law as reflected in UNCLOS, which provides the legal framework for the conservation and sustainable use of oceans and their resources, as recalled in paragraph 158 of The Future We Want.

Source: United Nations. Sustainable Development Goals Knowledge Platform.
https://sustainabledevelopment.un.org

4.15. Sustainable Development Goal 15

Sustainable Development Goal 15 aims to protect, restore and promote sustainable use of terrestrial ecosystems, sustainably manage forests, combat desertification, and halt and reverse land degradation and halt biodiversity loss (Table **6.15**). Protecting and preserving diverse forms of life on land requires focused efforts to protect and promote the conservation and sustainable use of land and other ecosystems. Goal 15 focuses specifically on managing forests sustainably, restoring degraded lands and combating desertification, and ending biodiversity loss.

Biodiversity or the variety of plant and animal life underpins ecosystem functioning and the provision of goods and services that are essential to human health and well-being [10, 11]. The conservation and the sustainable use of biodiversity can benefit human health by preserving ecosystem services and options for the future. Biodiversity, ecosystems, health and human activity are interlinked and interact in many ways [73]. For example, the variety of species provide nutrients and medicines; ecosystem functioning provides services such as water and air purification, pest and disease control and pollination; air and water pollution can lead to biodiversity loss and disease; and the excessive use of pharmaceuticals may release active ingredients to the environment and damage species and ecosystems. Both biodiversity and health can be damaged due to land-use change, habitat loss, overexploitation, pollution, invasive species, climate change and large-scale social and economic projects. A social justice perspective is needed to address the various dimensions of equity in the biodiversity and health dynamic because vulnerable groups (such as women and the poor) suffer disproportionately from biodiversity loss as they tend to be more reliant on ecosystem services and have less access to social protection mechanisms [73].

Damage to biodiversity and ecosystems of planet earth is not only due to human activities. Large scale destruction of forests and the environment has also been caused by unregulated actions and profit making motives of large international corporations and syndicates. According to a study conducted by the United Nations, the cost of pollution and other damage to the natural environment caused by the world's largest companies would take away one third of their profits, if they were held financially accountable to the damage.

According to United Nations data, between 1990 and 2015, the world's forest area diminished from 31.7% of the world's total land mass to 30.7% [11]. The loss was mainly attributable to the conversion of forest to other land uses. Owing to efforts to slow deforestation, such as planting and landscape restoration, the global net loss of forest area declined from 7.3 million hectares per year in the 1990s to 3.3 million hectares per year during the period from 2010 to 2015.

Table 6.15. Sustainable Development Goal 15 targets.

15.1
By 2020, ensure the conservation, restoration and sustainable use of terrestrial and inland freshwater ecosystems and their services, in particular forests, wetlands, mountains and drylands, in line with obligations under international agreements.
15.2
By 2020, promote the implementation of sustainable management of all types of forests, halt deforestation, restore degraded forests and substantially increase afforestation and reforestation globally.
15.3
By 2030, combat desertification, restore degraded land and soil, including land affected by desertification, drought and floods, and strive to achieve a land degradation-neutral world.
15.4
By 2030, ensure the conservation of mountain ecosystems, including their biodiversity, in order to enhance their capacity to provide benefits that are essential for sustainable development.
15.5
Take urgent and significant action to reduce the degradation of natural habitats, halt the loss of biodiversity and, by 2020, protect and prevent the extinction of threatened species.
15.6
Promote fair and equitable sharing of the benefits arising from the utilization of genetic resources and promote appropriate access to such resources, as internationally agreed.
15.7
Take urgent action to end poaching and trafficking of protected species of flora and fauna and address both demand and supply of illegal wildlife products.
15.8
By 2020, introduce measures to prevent the introduction and significantly reduce the impact of invasive alien species on land and water ecosystems and control or eradicate the priority species.
15.9
By 2020, integrate ecosystem and biodiversity values into national and local planning, development processes, poverty reduction strategies and accounts.
15.a
Mobilize and significantly increase financial resources from all sources to conserve and sustainably use biodiversity and ecosystems.
15.b
Mobilize significant resources from all sources and at all levels to finance sustainable forest management and provide adequate incentives to developing countries to advance such management, including for conservation and reforestation.
15.c
Enhance global support for efforts to combat poaching and trafficking of protected species, including by increasing the capacity of local communities to pursue sustainable livelihood opportunities.

Source: United Nations. Sustainable Development Goals Knowledge Platform.
https://sustainabledevelopment.un.org

To safeguard places that contribute significantly to global biodiversity, protected areas have been identified as key biodiversity areas. In 2014, 15.2% of the world's terrestrial and freshwater environments were covered by protected areas.

The percentage of terrestrial key biodiversity areas covered by protected areas has increased, about 3% from 2000 to 2016. Over the same period, the share of freshwater key biodiversity areas that are protected has increased from 13.8% to 16.6%.

The focus of Goal 15 on halting biodiversity loss comes at a critical time, since many animal species are at imminent risk of extinction. However, their decline can be prevented. For example extinction risks for vertebrate species have been reversed in five small island developing states (the Cook Islands, Fiji, Mauritius, Seychelles and Tonga) as a result of conservation efforts over the past several decades [10, 11]. Conservation efforts are undermined by poaching and the trafficking of wildlife. Since 1999, as many as 7000 species of animals and plants have been detected in illegal trade [11]. In 2014, bilateral official development assistance to support biodiversity amounted to US$ 7 billion, an increase of 16% in real terms over 2013.

To attain this goal, national plans need to be developed and implemented to ensure the conservation, restoration and sustainable management of terrestrial and inland freshwater ecosystems to halt deforestation and trafficking of protected species of flora and fauna.

4.16. Sustainable Development Goal 16

Sustainable Development Goal 16 is dedicated to provision of universal access to justice, building effective, accountable institutions and the promotion of peaceful and inclusive societies for sustainable development (Table **6.16**). Many countries, particularly in the developed world, have enjoyed peace and security in recent decades. But there are many countries in the developing world that experience prolonged armed conflict and civil unrest, often resulting in massive population displacements and humanitarian needs. These unstable situations render disadvantaged populations increasingly vulnerable to overcrowding, inadequate sanitation, insufficient food supply, and disruptions to health-care services. These factors interact synergistically to result in an increased incidence of NCDs as well as progression of existing disease, resulting in complications such as stroke.

People in many countries suffer from the lack of access to information, freedom of expression, justice and other fundamental freedoms. According to United Nations data, corruption, bribery, theft and tax evasion cost some US$ 1.26 trillion for developing countries per year. Alarmingly, judiciary and police are the institutions most affected by corruption, undermining confidence in state institutions [10, 11, 74].

Limited data from 19 countries indicated that the rate of prevalence of bribery is as high as 50% among citizens who had contact with public officials [11, 74]. The number of victims of intentional homicide was estimated at between 4.6 and 6.8 per 100 000 people in 2014. Worldwide, the proportion of people held in detention without sentencing was 30% in 2012–2014 [11, 74]. Only 35.5% of countries have national human rights institutions. A free press plays a key role in access to information and the protection of human rights. About 90 States have adopted laws on freedom of speech but the number of journalists killed has doubled from 65 in 2010 to 114 in 2015 [11, 74].

Table 6.16. Sustainable development goal 16 targets.

GOAL 16 TARGETS
16.1 Significantly reduce all forms of violence and related death rates everywhere.
16.2 End abuse, exploitation, trafficking and all forms of violence against and torture of children.
16.3 Promote the rule of law at the national and international levels and ensure equal access to justice for all.
16.4 By 2030, significantly reduce illicit financial and arms flows, strengthen the recovery and return of stolen assets and combat all forms of organized crime.
16.5 Substantially reduce corruption and bribery in all their forms.
16.6 Develop effective, accountable and transparent institutions at all levels.
16.7 Ensure responsive, inclusive, participatory and representative decision-making at all levels.
16.8 Broaden and strengthen the participation of developing countries in the institutions of global governance.
16.9 By 2030, provide legal identity for all, including birth registration.
16.10 Ensure public access to information and protect fundamental freedoms, in accordance with national legislation and international agreements.
16.a Strengthen relevant national institutions, including through international cooperation, for building capacity at all levels, in particular in developing countries, to prevent violence and combat terrorism and crime.
16.b Promote and enforce non-discriminatory laws and policies for sustainable development.

Source: United Nations. Sustainable Development Goals Knowledge Platform.
https://sustainabledevelopment.un.org

Human rights and accountability are relevant to the three strategic approaches required to address NCDs: prevention; health care; and monitoring [75, 76]. First, a human rights-based approach helps to go beyond the behavioural risk factors to consider underlying and root causes such as the enjoyment of a range of health-related human rights such as the rights to healthy food, information and education. Second, such an approach maps the various stakeholders involved in promoting or undermining actions to address NCDs. Within government, specific duty-holders identified will range across sectors such as agriculture, finance and taxation, education, recreation, media, transportation and urban planning. A range of other duty-bearers can be identified that have specific responsibilities. These may range from family members to multinational corporations, donors and the private sector, including the tobacco, food, sugar and alcohol industries. Under international human rights law, governments are under obligation to promote and protect human rights across all sectors, including the private sector, so that it acts in conformity with human rights. A human rights based-approach recognizes relationships in order to empower people to advocate for and claim their rights. Such an approach also encourages policy-makers and service providers to meet their responsibilities and obligations in creating more responsive public health and health-care systems. To address NCDs (stroke), policies and programmes are required that are designed to protect health and be responsive to the needs of the population as a result of established accountability.

Actions to attain Goal 16 indirectly strengthen country capacity to address NCDs (stroke) because legal, regulatory and governance reforms lie at the centre of multisectoral national NCD responses. Reducing exposure of populations to NCD risk factors cannot be achieved without government leadership and governance structures to implement and monitor public health laws, regulations and policies [18, 75, 76]. Stricter regulation of the private sector is required in order to align profit-driven business activities closely with public health goals. Legal and regulatory actions for the prevention and control of NCDs require observance of the rule of law, and a political leadership and a trained public health workforce that are impervious to corruption. In addition, key to the success of a national NCD response is the freedom of the press to inform and harness the drive of civil society organizations to create a social movement that influences and monitors the policy agenda of the government.

To attain this goal countries have to take action to protect fundamental freedoms, improve access to justice, end abuse, exploitation, trafficking, corruption, terrorism, organized crime and all forms of violence.

4.17. Sustainable Development Goal 17

Sustainable Development Goal 17 aims to strengthen the means of implementation and revitalize the global partnership for sustainable development (Table **6.17**). Achieving the 169 targets of the 2030 Agenda for Sustainable Development requires a strong global partnership that brings together multiple stakeholders, including governments, civil society, the private sector, media, communities, the United Nations system and other actors [77 - 81].

Weak capacity for collecting data and monitoring is a major obstacle to accountability of advancing the 2030 Agenda for Sustainable Development in developing countries. For example, in 2014, birth registration data were available for 183 out of 230 countries. Death registration data were available only for 157 countries [11].

Table 6.17. Sustainable development goal 17 targets.

Finance
17.1
Strengthen domestic resource mobilization, including through international support to developing countries, to improve domestic capacity for tax and other revenue collection.
17.2
Developed countries to implement fully their official development assistance commitments, including the commitment by many developed countries to achieve the target of 0.7 per cent of ODA/GNI to developing countries and 0.15 to 0.20 per cent of ODA/GNI to least-developed countries; ODA providers are encouraged to consider setting a target to provide at least 0.20 per cent of ODA/GNI to least-developed countries.
17.3
Mobilize additional financial resources for developing countries from multiple sources.
17.4
Assist developing countries in attaining long-term debt sustainability through coordinated policies aimed at fostering debt financing, debt relief and debt restructuring, as appropriate, and address the external debt of highly indebted poor countries to reduce debt distress
17.5
Adopt and implement investment promotion regimes for least-developed countries.
Technology
17.6
Enhance North–South, South–South and triangular regional and international cooperation on and access to science, technology and innovation and enhance knowledge sharing on mutually agreed terms, including through improved coordination among existing mechanisms, in particular at the United Nations level, and through a global technology facilitation mechanism.
17.7
Promote the development, transfer, dissemination and diffusion of environmentally sound technologies to developing countries on favourable terms, including on concessional and preferential terms, as mutually agreed.
17.8
Fully operationalize the technology bank and science, technology and innovation capacity-building mechanism for least-developed countries by 2017 and enhance the use of enabling technology, in particular information and communications technology.
Capacity-building
17.9
Enhance international support for implementing effective and targeted capacity-building in developing countries to support national plans to implement all the sustainable development goals, including through North-South, South-South and triangular cooperation.
Trade
17.10
Promote a universal, rules-based, open, non-discriminatory and equitable multilateral trading system under the World Trade Organization, including through the conclusion of negotiations under its Doha Development Agenda.
17.11
Significantly increase the exports of developing countries, in particular with a view to doubling the least-developed countries' share of global exports by 2020.

17.12
Realize timely implementation of duty-free and quota-free market access on a lasting basis for all least-developed countries, consistent with World Trade Organization decisions, including by ensuring that preferential rules of origin applicable to imports from least-developed countries are transparent and simple, and contribute to facilitating market access.
Systemic issues
Policy and institutional coherence
17.13
Enhance global macroeconomic stability, including through policy coordination and policy coherence.
17.14
Enhance policy coherence for sustainable development.
17.15
Respect each country's policy space and leadership to establish and implement policies for poverty eradication and sustainable development.
Multistakeholder partnerships
17.16
Enhance the global partnership for sustainable development, complemented by multistakeholder partnerships that mobilize and share knowledge, expertise, technology and financial resources, to support the achievement of the sustainable development goals in all countries, in particular developing countries.
17.17
Encourage and promote effective public, public-private and civil society partnerships, building on the experience and resourcing strategies of partnerships.
Data, monitoring and accountability
17.18
By 2020, enhance capacity-building support to developing countries, including for least-developed countries and small island developing States, to increase significantly the availability of high-quality, timely and reliable data disaggregated by income, gender, age, race, ethnicity, migratory status, disability, geographic location and other characteristics relevant in national contexts.
17.19
By 2030, build on existing initiatives to develop measurements of progress on sustainable development that complement gross domestic product, and support statistical capacity-building in developing countries.

GNI = gross national income
ODA = official development assistance
Source: United Nations. Sustainable Development Goals Knowledge Platform.
https://sustainabledevelopment.un.org

Only 58% of developing countries with available data have birth registration coverage of 90% or more. Registering all births and deaths is a first step in safeguarding individual rights and access to justice.

Progress in sustainable development in low- and middle-income countries is also hampered by inadequate access to Internet services. In 2015, fixed-broadband penetration had reached to 29% in the developed regions, but only 0.5% in the least-developed countries [11]. In developing regions, one third of the population is online *versus* 1 in 10 people in the least-developed countries.

Mobilizing resources and enhancing support to developing countries are important to equitable progress for all. Developed countries have made commitments to meet the United Nations target for official development assistance of 0.7% of official development assistance/gross national income to developing countries and 0.15–0.20% to least-developed countries [10, 11, 82]. In 2015, net official development assistance from member countries of the Development Assistance Committee of the Organisation for Economic Co-operation and Development totalled US$ 131.6 billion. Only seven countries met the United Nations target for official development assistance of 0.7% of gross national income in 2015, in Denmark, Luxembourg, the Netherlands, Norway, Sweden, the United Arab Emirates and the United Kingdom.

CONCLUDING REMARKS

The Sustainable Development Goals recognize the negative and positive links between health, its determinants and sustainable development. If all countries are to benefit from the transformational ambition of the sustainable development agenda, developing countries need to receive international support for strengthening capacity particularly to ensure policy coherence for sustainable development and monitoring progress. Ensuring policy coherence across different sectors of the Government is a challenging task. It requires multisectoral collaboration and multi stakeholder understanding of the trade-offs and potential synergies across economic growth, trade, investment, agriculture, health and NCDs (stroke), education, the environment and development co-operation. The 17 Sustainable Development Goals with the monitoring framework provide a unifying platform for progressive realization of this challenging task.

CONFLICT OF INTEREST

The author declares no conflict of interest, financial or otherwise.

ACKNOWLEDGEMENTS

Ms AvisAnne Julien is thanked for copy-editing.

REFERENCES

[1]   The millennium development goals report 2014 2014. Available at: http://www.un.org/ millenniumgoals/2014%20MDG%20report/MDG%202014%20English%20web.pdf

[2]   Kenny C, Sumner A. More money or more development: What have the MDGs achieved? Working Paper No 278, Center for Global Development: Washington DC 2011.

[3]   Copestake J, Williams R. Political-economy analysis, aid effectiveness and the art of development management. Dev Policy Rev 2014; 32: 133-53.
        [http://dx.doi.org/10.1111/dpr.12047]

[4]   The millennium development goals report 2014 2015. Available at: http://www.un.org/ millenniumgoals/2015_MDG_Report/pdf/MDG%202015%20rev%20(July%201).pdf

[5]   A new global partnership: eradicate poverty and transform economies through sustainable development Report of the High-level Panel of Eminent Persons on the Post-2015 Development Agenda. New York: United Nations 2013.

[6]   Resolution A/RES/66/288. The future we want. Adopted by the Sixty-sixth United Nations General Assembly, New York 2012.

[7]   The right to health is established as a fundamental right of every human being in Article 1 of the World Health Organization Constitution 1948. Available at: http://www.who.int/governance/ eb/who_constitution_en.pdf

[8]   Hill PS, Buse K, Brolan CE, Ooms G. How can health remain central post-2015 in a sustainable development paradigm? Global Health 2014; 10: 18.
[http://dx.doi.org/10.1186/1744-8603-10-18] [PMID: 24708779]

[9]   A68/17. Report of the Secretariat. Contributing to social and economic development: sustainable action across sectors to improve health and health equity (follow-up of the 8th Global Conference on Health Promotion). Sixty-eighth World Health Assembly, provisional agenda item 145, Geneva 2015.

[10]   Report of the united nations secretary-general. E/2016/75. Progress towards the sustainable development goals Available at: http://unstats.un.org/sdgs/files/report/ 2016/secretary-general-s-g-report-2016--EN.pdf

[11]   Sustainable development goals knowledge platform. Available at: https://sustainabledevelopment. un.org

[12]   Kwan GF, Mayosi BM, Mocumbi AO, *et al.* Endemic cardiovascular diseases of the poorest billion. Circulation 2016; 133(24): 2561-75.
[http://dx.doi.org/10.1161/CIRCULATIONAHA.116.008731] [PMID: 27297348]

[13]   Mendis S, Banerjee A. Cardiovascular disease, equity and social determinants. Equity, social determinants and public health programmes. □Geneva: World Health Organization 2010.

[14]   Garbusinski JM, van der Sande MA, Bartholome EJ, *et al.* Stroke presentation and outcome in developing countries: a prospective study in the Gambia Stroke 2005; 36: 1388-93.

[15]   Walker RW, McLarty DG, Kitange HM, *et al.* Stroke mortality in urban and rural Tanzania. Adult morbidity and mortality project. Lancet 2000; 355(9216): 1684-7.
[http://dx.doi.org/10.1016/S0140-6736(00)02240-6] [PMID: 10905244]

[16]   Walker RW, Rolfe M, Kelly PJ, George MO, James OF. Mortality and recovery after stroke in the Gambia. Stroke 2003; 34(7): 1604-9.
[http://dx.doi.org/10.1161/01.STR.0000077943.63718.67] [PMID: 12817107]

[17]   Pandian JD, Srikanth V, Read SJ, Thrift AG. Poverty and stroke in India: a time to act. Stroke 2007; 38(11): 3063-9.
[http://dx.doi.org/10.1161/STROKEAHA.107.496869] [PMID: 17954905]

[18]   Global status report on noncommunicable diseases 2014. Geneva: World Health Organization 2014.

[19]   Barker DJ, Osmond C, Law CM. The intrauterine and early postnatal origins of cardiovascular disease and chronic bronchitis. J Epidemiol Community Health 1989; 43(3): 237-40.
[http://dx.doi.org/10.1136/jech.43.3.237] [PMID: 2607302]

[20]   Godfrey KM, Gluckman PD, Hanson MA. Developmental origins of metabolic disease: life course and intergenerational perspectives. Trends Endocrinol Metab 2010; 21(4): 199-205.
[http://dx.doi.org/10.1016/j.tem.2009.12.008] [PMID: 20080045]

[21]   Vickers MH, Breier BH, Cutfield WS, Hofman PL, Gluckman PD. Fetal origins of hyperphagia, obesity, and hypertension and postnatal amplification by hypercaloric nutrition. Am J Physiol Endocrinol Metab 2000; 279(1): E83-7.
[PMID: 10893326]

[22]   Burdge GC, Hanson MA, Slater-Jefferies JL, Lillycrop KA. Epigenetic regulation of transcription: a mechanism for inducing variations in phenotype (fetal programming) by differences in nutrition during early life? Br J Nutr 2007; 97(6): 1036-46.
       [http://dx.doi.org/10.1017/S0007114507682920] [PMID: 17381976]

[23]   Waterland RA, Jirtle RL. Transposable elements: targets for early nutritional effects on epigenetic gene regulation. Mol Cell Biol 2003; 23(15): 5293-300.
       [http://dx.doi.org/10.1128/MCB.23.15.5293-5300.2003] [PMID: 12861015]

[24]   Unpublished work for the report using methods from: WHO global report on trends in tobacco smoking 2000–2025 2015. Available at: http://www. who.int/tobacco/publications/surveillance/reportontrendstobaccosmoking/en/

[25]   Burden of disease from the joint effects of household and ambient air pollution for 2012 2014. Available at: http://www.who.int/phe/health_topics/outdoorair/databases/AP_jointeffect_BoD_results_March2014.pdf

[26]   Global Health Observatory data: household air pollution Available at: http://www.who.int/gho/phe/indoor_air_pollution/en/

[27]   van Donkelaar A, Martin RV, Brauer M, Boys BL. Use of satellite observations for long-term exposure assessment of global concentrations of fine particulate matter. Environ Health Perspect 2015; 123(2): 135-43.
       [PMID: 25343779]

[28]   Indoor air quality guidelines: household fuel combustion 2014. Available at: http://www.who.int/indoorair/guidelines/hhfc/en/

[29]   Package of essential noncommunicable (PEN) disease interventions for primary health care in low-resource settings 2010. Available at: http://www.who.int/nmh/publications/essential_ncd_interventions_lr_settings.pdf

[30]   Implementation tools Package of essential noncommunicable (PEN) disease interventions for primary health care in low-resource settings 2013. Available at: http://apps.who.int/iris/bitstream/10665/133525/1/9789241506557_eng.pdf

[31]   Global action plan for the prevention and control of noncommunicable diseases 2013-2020 2013. Available at: http://apps.who. int/iris/bitstream/10665/94384/1/9789241506236_ eng.pdf?ua=1

[32]   Tracking universal health coverage: first global monitoring report. Joint WHO/World Bank Group report 2015.

[33]   A/70/320 Report of the Secretary-General on the follow-up to and implementation of the outcomes of the third United Nations International Conference on Financing for Development 2015. Available at: http://www.un.org/ga/search/view_doc.asp?symbol=A/70/320

[34]   MDG 2: Achieve universal primary education. MDG Monitor Available at: www.mdgmonitor.org/mdg-2-achieve-universal-primary-education/

[35]   Women constitutional database. UN. New York: United Nations 2014.

[36]   Women UN. Progress of the World's Women 2015–2016 Transforming economies, realizing rights. NewYork: United Nations 2015.

[37]   Women in national parliaments. New York: Inter-Parliamentary Union 2015.

[38]   Global and regional estimates of violence against women: prevalence and health effects of intimate partner violence and non-partner sexual violence. Geneva: World Health Organization 2013.

[39]   Appelros P, Stegmayr B, Terént A. Sex differences in stroke epidemiology: a systematic review. Stroke 2009; 40(4): 1082-90.
       [http://dx.doi.org/10.1161/STROKEAHA.108.540781] [PMID: 19211488]

[40]   Delbari A, Keyghobadi F, Momtaz YA, *et al.* Sex differences in stroke: a socioeconomic perspective. Clin Interv Aging 2016; 11: 1207-12.
[http://dx.doi.org/10.2147/CIA.S113302] [PMID: 27660426]

[41]   Haast RA, Gustafson DR, Kiliaan AJ. Sex differences in stroke. J Cereb Blood Flow Metab 2012; 32(12): 2100-7.
[http://dx.doi.org/10.1038/jcbfm.2012.141] [PMID: 23032484]

[42]   Das SK, Banerjee TK, Biswas A, *et al.* A prospective community-based study of stroke in Kolkata, India. Stroke 2007; 38(3): 906-10.
[http://dx.doi.org/10.1161/01.STR.0000258111.00319.58] [PMID: 17272773]

[43]   Reeves MJ, Bushnell CD, Howard G, *et al.* Sex differences in stroke: epidemiology, clinical presentation, medical care, and outcomes. Lancet Neurol 2008; 7(10): 915-26.
[http://dx.doi.org/10.1016/S1474-4422(08)70193-5] [PMID: 18722812]

[44]   Momtaz YA, Haron SA, Ibrahim R, Hamid TA. Social embeddedness as a mechanism for linking social cohesion to well-being among older adults: moderating effect of gender. Clin Interv Aging 2014; 9: 863-70.
[http://dx.doi.org/10.2147/CIA.S62205] [PMID: 24904206]

[45]   Turtzo LC, McCullough LD. Sex differences in stroke. Cerebrovasc Dis 2008; 26(5): 462-74.
[http://dx.doi.org/10.1159/000155983] [PMID: 18810232]

[46]   Bushnell C, McCullough LD, Awad IA, *et al.* Guidelines for the prevention of stroke in women: a statement for healthcare professionals from the American Heart Association/American Stroke Association. Stroke 2014; 45(5): 1545-88.
[http://dx.doi.org/10.1161/01.str.0000442009.06663.48] [PMID: 24503673]

[47]   Smith MA, Lisabeth LD, Bonikowski F, Morgenstern LB. The role of ethnicity, sex, and language on delay to hospital arrival for acute ischemic stroke. Stroke 2010; 41(5): 905-9.
[http://dx.doi.org/10.1161/STROKEAHA.110.578112] [PMID: 20339124]

[48]   Williams JE, Chimowitz MI, Cotsonis GA, Lynn MJ, Waddy SP. Gender differences in outcomes among patients with symptomatic intracranial arterial stenosis. Stroke 2007; 38(7): 2055-62.
[http://dx.doi.org/10.1161/STROKEAHA.107.482240] [PMID: 17540969]

[49]   Glader E-L, Stegmayr B, Norrving B, *et al.* Sex differences in management and outcome after stroke: a Swedish national perspective. Stroke 2003; 34(8): 1970-5.
[http://dx.doi.org/10.1161/01.STR.0000083534.81284.C5] [PMID: 12855818]

[50]   Persky RW, Turtzo LC, McCullough LD. Stroke in women: disparities and outcomes. Curr Cardiol Rep 2010; 12(1): 6-13.
[http://dx.doi.org/10.1007/s11886-009-0080-2] [PMID: 20425178]

[51]   Lisabeth LD, Reeves MJ, Baek J, *et al.* Factors influencing **sex** differences in poststroke functional outcome. Stroke 2015; 46(3): 860-3.
[http://dx.doi.org/10.1161/STROKEAHA.114.007985] [PMID: 25633999]

[52]   Gleick PH. Water and conflict. Int Secur 1993; 18(1): 79-112.
[http://dx.doi.org/10.2307/2539033]

[53]   Mücke S, Grotemeyer KH, Stahlhut L, Husstedt IW, Evers S. The influence of fluid intake on stroke recurrence--a prospective study. J Neurol Sci 2012; 315(1-2): 82-5. [Epub 6 December 2011].
[http://dx.doi.org/10.1016/j.jns.2011.11.024] [PMID: 22169398]

[54]   Levy BS, Sidel VW. Water rights and water fights: preventing and resolving conflicts before they boil over. Am J Public Health 2011; 101(5): 778-80.
[http://dx.doi.org/10.2105/AJPH.2010.194670] [PMID: 21421949]

[55]   Cairncross S, Bartram J, Cumming O, Brocklehurst C. Hygiene, sanitation, and water: what needs to be done? PLoS Med 2010; 7(11): e1000365.

[http://dx.doi.org/10.1371/journal.pmed.1000365] [PMID: 21125019]

[56]   Anderson BA, Romani JH, Phillips H, Wentzel M, Tlabela K. Exploring environmental perceptions, behaviors and awareness: water and water pollution in South Africa. Popul Environ 2007; 28: 133-61.
[http://dx.doi.org/10.1007/s11111-007-0038-5]

[57]   Energy - United Nations Sustainable Development. Available at: http://www.un.org/sustainable development/energy/

[58]   Frank Julio Health and the economy: a vital relationship. OECD Observer 2004. Available at: http://oecdobserver.org/news/archivestory.php/aid/1241/Health_and_the_economy:_A_vital_relations hip_.html

[59]   Cities for health. Kobe: WHO and Metropolis 2014.

[60]   Global report on urban health: equitable healthier cities for sustainable development. Geneva: World Health Organization and UN-Habitat 2016.

[61]   Health in the green economy: health co-benefits of climate change mitigation – housing sector. Geneva: World Health Organization 2011.

[62]   Health in the green economy: health co-benefits of climate change mitigation – transport sector. Geneva: World Health Organization 2011.

[63]   Global waste trade Available at: https://en.wikipedia.org/wiki/Global_waste_trade#Impacts_of_the_ global_waste_trade

[64]   The Basel convention on the control of transboundary movements of hazardous wastes and their disposal Available at: http://www.basel.int

[65]   The Stockholm Convention on persistent organic pollutants Available at: http://chm.pops.int/ TheConvention/Overview/tabid/3351/

[66]   The Rotterdam convention. Available at: http://www.pic.int

[67]   United Nations framework convention on climate change. 1992. Available at: http://unfccc. int/files/essential_background/background_publications_htmlpdf/application/pdf/conveng.pdf

[68]   Pachauri RK, Reisinger A. Core writing team. Contribution of working groups I, II and III to the fourth assessment report of the intergovernmental panel on climate change. Intergovernmental panel on climate change Available at: http://www.ipcc.ch/publications_and_data/ar4/syr/en/spm.html

[69]   United Nations. Paris agreement 2015. Available at: http://unfccc.int/files/essential_background/ convention/application/pdf/english_paris_agreement.pdf

[70]   New policy brief on climate and noncommunicable diseases 2016. Available at: https://ncdalliance.org/news-events/news/new-policy-brief-on-climate-cha-ge-and-ncds-launched-today

[71]   United Nations development programme. Sustainable Development Goal 14 Life below water Available   at: http://www.undp.org/content/undp/en/home/sustainable-development-goals/goal-14-life-below-water. html

[72]   Lamborg CH, Hammerschmidt CR, Bowman KL, *et al.* A global ocean inventory of anthropogenic mercury based on water column measurements. Nature 2014; 512(7512): 65-8.
[http://dx.doi.org/10.1038/nature13563] [PMID: 25100482]

[73]   Connecting global priorities: biodiversity and human health. Geneva: World Health Organization and secretariat of the convention on biological diversity 2015. Available at: https://www.cbd.int/health/SOK-biodiversity-en.pdf

[74]   Sustainable development goals. 17 Goals to transform our world Available at: http://www.un.org/sustainabledevelopment/peace-justice/

[75] Nygren-krug H. A human rights-based approach to noncommunicable diseases Available at: http://lawexplores.com/a-human-rights-based-approach-to-non-communicable-diseases/

[76] Magnusson RS, Patterson D. The role of law and governance reform in the global response to non-communicable diseases. Global Health 2014; 10: 44.
[http://dx.doi.org/10.1186/1744-8603-10-44] [PMID: 24903332]

[77] A new global partnership: eradicate poverty and transform economies through sustainable development Report of the high-level panel of eminent persons on the post-2015 development agenda. New York: United Nations 2013.

[78] Buse K, Hawkes S. Health post-2015: evidence and power. Lancet 2014; 383(9918): 678-9.
[http://dx.doi.org/10.1016/S0140-6736(13)61945-5] [PMID: 24055453]

[79] The future we want: outcome document adopted at Rio+20 2013. Available at: http://www.un.org/en/sustainablefuture/

[80] Frenk J, Gómez-Dantés O, Moon S. From sovereignty to solidarity: a renewed concept of global health for an era of complex interdependence. Lancet 2014; 383(9911): 94-7.
[http://dx.doi.org/10.1016/S0140-6736(13)62561-1] [PMID: 24388312]

[81] Jamison DT, Summers LH, Alleyne G, *et al.* Global health 2035: a world converging within a generation. Lancet 2013; 382(9908): 1898-955.
[http://dx.doi.org/10.1016/S0140-6736(13)62105-4] [PMID: 24309475]

[82] Beyond 2015: towards a comprehensive and integrated approach to financing poverty eradication and sustainable development 2013. Available at: http://ec.europa.eu/europeaid/what/ development-policies/financing_for_development/documents/accountability-report-2013/accountabili-y-report-2013-01_en.pdf

CHAPTER 7

Economic and Societal Costs of Stroke

Shanthi Mendis[*]

Geneva Learning Foundation, Former Senior Adviser World Health Organization, Geneva, Switzerland

Abstract: Direct and indirect costs of stroke (NCDs) adversely impact macroeconomic productivity and national and household income pose a significant financial burden on health-care budgets. The estimated global economic loss due to cardiovascular disease (stroke and heart disease) has been estimated at US$ 863.5 billion in 2010. It is estimated to increase by 22% and to US$ 1.04 billion in 2030. For the period 2011–2025, the cumulative lost output in low- and middle-income countries associated with cardiovascular disease (stroke and heart disease) is projected at more than US$ 3.76 trillion. The total cost of implementing a set of very cost effective interventions for prevention and management of stroke across all low- and middle-income countries for the period 2011–2025, is estimated at only US$ 170 billion. This amounts to an annual per person investment of under US$ 1 in low-income countries, US$ 1.50 in lower-middle-income countries and US$ 3 in upper-middle-income countries.

Keywords: Cardiovascular disease, Cost-effective interventions, Direct costs, Economic burden, Household income, Indirect costs, Low- and middle-income countries, Macroeconomic productivity, National income, Stroke.

INTRODUCTION

This chapter addresses the following questions.

1. What is the magnitude of the economic burden of stroke globally?
2. What is the projected cost of stroke for low and middle income countries?
3. What is the impact of stroke on macroeconomic productivity?
4. What is known about the indirect costs of stroke?
5. What is known about the direct costs of stroke?
6. How do stroke costs impact on national health care expenditure?
7. What is the cost of treating an acute stroke?
8. What is the cost of atrial fibrillation related stroke?
9. What are the hospital costs of stroke based on population studies?

[*] **Corresponding author Shanthi Mendis:** Geneva Learning Foundation, Geneva, Switzerland; Tel/Fax: 0041227880311; E-mail: prof.shanthi.mendis@gmail.com

Shanthi Mendis (Ed.)

10. What are the social costs and consequences of stroke?
11. What are the economic consequences of stroke on households?

1. WHAT IS THE MAGNITUDE OF THE ECONOMIC BURDEN OF STROKE GLOBALLY?

Stroke (NCDs) adversely affect economic growth through several pathways [1 - 7]. First, stroke exerts a negative macroeconomic impact through labour and productivity losses of affected people and their caregivers. Second, it drives up national health-care spending due to direct costs of medical care; and third, stroke increases out-of-pocket expenditures for households and contributes to impoverishment.

A study conducted by the World Economic Forum and the Harvard School of Public Health used three distinct approaches to compute the global economic burden of stroke (NCDs) for the period 2011–2030: (i) the standard cost of illness method; (ii) macroeconomic simulation; and (iii) the value of a statistical life [6]. These methods yielded results that are not comparable. Nevertheless, the estimates of this study give a sense of the current staggering costs and the growing economic burden of stroke (NCDs). To obtain a more reliable sense of the global cost of stroke more data are required particularly from low and middle income countries.

The cost of illness method looks at the cost of disease as the sum of several categories of direct and indirect costs. The estimated economic loss due to cardiovascular disease (stroke and heart disease), using this method was US$ 863.5 billion in 2010 (Table **7.1**) (an average per person cost of US$ 125) [6]. This loss is estimated to increase by 22% and to US$ 1.04 billion in 2030.

Table 7.1. Costs attributable to stroke and heart disease (cardiovascular diseases) in 2010 by WHO region. Source: Adapted from Bloom, D.E., Cafiero, E.T., Jané-Llopis, E., Abrahams-Gessel, S., Bloom, L.R., Fathima, S., Feigl, A.B., Gaziano, T., Mowafi, M., Pandya, A., Prettner, K., Rosenberg, L., Seligman, B., Stein, A.Z., & Weinstein, C. (2011). The Global Economic Burden of Noncommunicable Diseases. Geneva: World Economic Forum.

WHO Region	Total Costs (Including Productivity Costs) Billions of US$
Africa	11.6
Americas	303.1
Eastern Mediterranean	18.3
Europe	392.6
South East Asia	30.7
Western Pacific	107.1

(Table 7.1) contd.....

WHO Region	Total Costs (Including Productivity Costs) Billions of US$
Total	863.5

Overall, the cost for cardiovascular disease could be as high as US$ 20 trillion over the 20-year period 2011–2030. In 2010, about US$ 474 billion (55%) was due to direct health-care costs and the remainder (45%) to productivity loss due to disability and premature death or time loss from work due to sickness [6].

The economic growth approach estimates the projected impact of NCDs on total economic output (GDP) by taking into account how these diseases deplete labour and capital. Applying this approach over this 20-year period, the estimated loss due to cardiovascular disease (stroke and heart disease), was US$ 15.6 trillion (Table **7.2**) [6].

Table 7.2. Economic burden of cardiovascular diseases (stroke and heart disease) using macroeconomic simulation approach (trillions of US$ 2010) Source: Adapted from Bloom, D.E., Cafiero, E.T., Jané-Llopis, E., Abrahams-Gessel, S., Bloom, L.R., Fathima, S., Feigl, A.B., Gaziano, T., Mowafi, M., Pandya, A., Prettner, K., Rosenberg, L., Seligman, B., Stein, A.Z., & Weinstein, C. (2011). The Global Economic Burden of Noncommunicable Diseases. Geneva: World Economic Forum.

Country Income Group	Cardiovascular Diseases
High income	8.5
Upper-middle income	4.8
Lower-middle	2.0
Low	0.3
World	15.6

The value of the statistical life method reflects a population's willingness to pay to reduce the risk of disability or death associated with NCDs. Using this approach, the estimated loss from cardiovascular disease (stroke and heart disease), was US$ 8.3 trillion in 2010, increasing to US$ 15.8 trillion in 2030 [6]. Cardiovascular disease accounted for 33% of the lost output due to NCDs and mental health. The high-income countries bear the highest absolute burden of the lost output followed by upper-middle-income, lower-middle-income and low-income countries. By 2030, the upper-middle-income countries will take on a much bigger share of the economic burden due to the size and growth of their income and ageing of their populations, which are larger than those of high-income countries.

2. WHAT IS THE PROJECTED COST OF STROKE IN LOW- AND MIDDLE-INCOME COUNTRIES?

To estimate the costs of stroke accurately, population-based studies with long-term follow-up are needed, reporting direct and indirect costs in unselected hospital- and community-treated patients with first-ever and recurrent stroke events. There is a lack of such comprehensive data for low- and middle-income countries. A part of the economic burden study carried out by the World Economic Forum and the Harvard School of Public Health assessed the economic losses associated with NCDs (includes stroke), focusing the analysis on low- and middle-income countries, which account for 84% of the world's population and 83% of the global NCD burden [7]. For the period 2011–2025, the cumulative lost output in low- and middle-income countries associated with the four major NCD conditions (cardiovascular disease, cancer, diabetes and chronic respiratory disease) was projected at more than US$ 7 trillion [7]. The annual loss of approximately US$ 500 billion amounted to roughly 4% of GDP for low- and middle-income countries in 2010. In every income group, estimated losses from NCDs are greater than public spending on health, assuming that inflation-adjusted levels of such spending remain at their 2009 levels for the period 2011–2025. Over the same period, the cumulative lost output in low- and middle-income countries associated with cardiovascular disease (stroke and heart disease), is projected at more than US$ 3.76 trillion. The total economic burden is higher in middle-income countries (US$ 3.59 trillion), in part because the value of lost earnings is high in this group of countries and in part because the total population includes China and India and is much higher than that of low-income countries.

A range of interventions for prevention and control of stroke (NCDs) exists [1]. In all countries, choices have to be made about which of these interventions are prioritized for implementation because there are other competing health issues and resources for health are limited [1, 8]. In preparation for the 2011 United Nations High-level Meeting on Noncommunicable Diseases, WHO identified a set of evidence-based "best buy" interventions that are not only very cost effective, but also feasible to implement within the constraints of the low- and middle-income country health systems [9]. The total cost of implementing the full set of "best buy" interventions across all low- and middle-income countries during 2011–2025 is estimated at US$ 170 billion, at an average of US$ 11.4 billion per year. This amounts to an annual per person investment of under US$ 1 in low-income countries, US$ 1.50 in lower-middle-income and US$ 3 in upper-middl--income countries. When the cost of such action is considered in terms of overall health spending, they amount to a small fraction of total health spending – 4% in low-income countries, 2% in lower-middle-income countries and less than 1% in upper-middle-income countries. Population-based measures for reducing tobacco and harmful alcohol use, as well as unhealthy diet and physical inactivity, are estimated to cost US\$ 2 billion per year for all low- and middle-income countries, which in fact translates to less than US\$ 0.40 per person.

3. WHAT IS THE IMPACT OF STROKE ON MACROECONOMIC PRODUCTIVITY?

Measures of productivity impact reported in studies include disability-adjusted life- years, labour market participation, return to work, absenteeism, change in hours worked, and medical or sickness leave. Most studies focus on the direct impact on the patient, but a minority also examined the impact on caregivers and spouses.

Although 82% of the stroke (NCD) burden is in low- and middle-income countries, the vast majority of studies (96%) investigating the macroeconomic impact of stroke are from high-income countries [3]. Studies from low-income countries are limited to Argentina, Brazil, Islamic Republic of Iran, Kenya, South Africa and the United Republic of Tanzania.

In Spain, stroke accounted for 3.5% of all disability-adjusted life years (DALYs) and the loss of 418 052 DALYs [10, 11]. This accounts for 1113 DALYs per 100 000 population (men: 1197 and women: 1033) and 3912 per 100 000 in those over age 65 (men: 4427 and women: 2033). A study from Kenya reported a rate of 166 DALYs per 100 000 person-years observed [3]. In Western Australia, the average annual stroke-attributable DALY count was an estimated 26 315 for men and 30 918 for women [12]. According to WHO definition, one DALY can be thought of as one lost year of "healthy" life. The sum of these DALYs across the population, or the burden of disease, can be thought of as a measurement of the gap between current health status and an ideal health situation where the entire population lives to an advanced age, free of disease and disability.

Even in settings with universal health coverage, up to 16% of patients die within the first 30 days after their stroke [13], and within 12months after the stroke event nearly 55% die or experience severe consequences [14]. About one half of survivors are left with permanent disabilities and have significant needs for rehabilitation [15].

There are considerable differences in costs between countries from productivity loss due to stroke [3]. Productivity losses in the Republic of Korea were 68% higher for a severe stroke among men (US\$ 537 724) than women (US\$ 171 157) [16]. A prospective surveillance study from the United Republic of Tanzania reported a mean costs of productivity loss of US\$ 213 on average, and these losses were most acutely experienced by those in higher skill roles [17]. The impact of stroke on return to work has been studied [18 - 20]. In Nigeria, 55% went back to work at a mean of 19.5 months after stroke. A report from the United Kingdom found that 47% were not in employment one year after stroke [20].

Since stroke often results in permanent disability and recurrences are common, costs sustained by patients suffering stroke at an earlier age would be greater compared to those of patients who suffered a stroke later in life. With the age distribution of stroke patients shifting towards younger ages, the future economic burden imposed by stroke is set to increase [21 - 24]. Further, due to improved stroke survival, the prevalence of stroke survivors within the working-age group is bound to increase. Based on available data, about 20% of stroke victims are in the working-age group [25]. Stroke in the working-age group causes a high economic burden due to direct costs of medical care as well as indirect costs associated with lost productivity [25 - 30].

Total mortality-related lifetime productivity loss from stroke cost the Korean economy 200.7, 81.9 and 16.4 million Korean won (1200 KRW is approximately equal to one US$ 1) for men who suffered a first stroke at age 45, 55 and 65 years, respectively, and 75.7, 39.2 and 19.3 million KRW for women at the same ages, respectively. While stroke occurring among Koreans aged 45–64 accounted for only 30% of the total disease incidence, this age group incurred 75% of the total national lifetime costs of stroke [16]. Lifetime costs of stroke are greater among men than women due to greater indirect costs [31].

There is also likely to be a differential impact of stroke on economic productivity in high-income and low- and middle-income countries because case fatality and disability rates are higher in low- and middle-income countries compared to high-income countries [32 - 36]. For instance, in the hospital-based INTERSTROKE study, the one-month case fatality rate for stroke was 22% in the WHO African Region [36].

The rates of full return to work one year after onset of stroke depends on the type and severity of stroke and varies from 35% to 62% in different studies [37 - 43]. These differences in return to work rates among different studies may be explained by differences in health-care systems, type of patients and study design. Return to work after stroke is an important outcome in stroke rehabilitation [43 - 46]. Promoting early return to work after stroke has individual benefits and also helps to reduce indirect costs associated with lost productivity [47].

Productivity loss often extends beyond the stroke survivor to caregivers. Many stroke survivors are unable perform simple activities, which exerts a considerable burden on informal caregivers. Depending on the stroke survivors' disability and nursing home coverage, informal caregivers experience varying degrees of overall work restriction, absenteeism and presenteeism. In one study, the mean total lost-productivity cost per employed caregiver was US$ 835 per month (>US$ 10 000 per year; 72% attributable to presenteeism) [48].

4. WHAT IS KNOWN ABOUT THE INDIRECT COSTS OF STROKE?

Indirect costs include productivity loss due to morbidity and mortality and costs of informal caregiving usually provided by unpaid family members. Studies focusing on indirect costs have investigated productivity losses and the cost of informal caregiving. Two approaches have been used for estimating the productivity loss [16, 49, 50]. The human capital approach estimates forgone earnings due to stroke as the productivity loss. The friction approach estimates the cost associated with the substitution of workers, including productivity losses due to replacement of workers or the training costs of new employees, as the productivity loss. The cost of informal caregiving has been estimated using two approaches [50]. The opportunity cost approach uses the value of each activity that informal caregivers sacrifice in order to provide informal care. The replacement approach assumes that an informal caregiver substitutes for a paid caregiver who would have provided the same type of caregiving services.

A recent review of 31 studies reported that indirect costs of stroke varied from 3% to 71% (median 32%) of the total cost of a stroke event [51]. Among the 31 studies reviewed, 19 were from European countries, 4 from Oceania, and 1 each from Canada and Thailand. The level of indirect cost depended on the length of study periods, methods, study design, type of stroke and cost components. Research on indirect cost of stroke in developing countries was lacking. Among the 31 studies reviewed, only one study was from a developing country. Some components of indirect cost, such as informal caregiving cost, are particularly important in developing countries as often organized care facilities or nursing home services for stroke survivors are lacking in these countries. As such, studies on informal caregiving in developing countries have public health significance in improving the quality of life for stroke patients.

Several cost of illness studies reported per-patient indirect costs. The follow-up period ranged from six months to a lifetime. In 2012 US dollars, the lowest per-patient indirect cost among 1-year follow-up studies was US$ 2960 in a German study, which did not include informal caregiving costs [52]. Lifetime follow-up costs for all types of stroke were US$ 22 243 per male and US$ 11 765 per female in a Swedish study, which did not include informal caregiving cost [53]. Lifetime follow-up costs in a study on haemorrhagic stroke in Spain, which included informal caregiving cost, was US$ 54 067 per patient [54]. Informal caregiving cost in this study was around 80% of the total indirect cost. The proportion of total cost that was represented by indirect cost for cost of illness studies ranged from a low of 3% for ischaemic stroke in a study from Australia [55] to a high of 71% in two studies, one from Spain [56] and the other from the United States [57].

Among studies that were confined to indirect costs several provided a per-patient estimate of the annual cost of informal caregiving. These costs ranged from US$ 904–1453 in a study from Thailand [58] to US$ 16 687–23 451 in a study from the Netherlands [50]. The annual morbidity cost in Sweden was estimated at US$ 14 963 per patient in 2006. The annual per-patient cost in the Thai study (US$ 904–1453) was much lower than the estimates from Western countries, which can be partly explained by the lower wages in Thailand.

The proportion of total cost represented by indirect cost ranged from 14% to 25% in Sweden [53, 59, 60], 3% to 10% in Australia and 6% to 9% [61] in New Zealand [62]. In a national-level United States study that focused entirely on indirect costs, annual cost of informal caregiving for elderly stroke patients was estimated at US$ 8.4 billion in 1993 [63]. In another study limited to the state of California, the annual cost of lost productivity associated with stroke mortality was reported at US$ 1.8 billion in 1991 [64]. Brown and colleagues estimated that indirect cost of ischaemic stroke (in 2012 US dollars) was US$ 1384 billion and indirect costs would account for 53% of the total costs of ischaemic stroke for the period of 2005–2050 [27]. More recently, Heidenreich and coworkers predicted that annual indirect cost (in 2012 US dollars) will increase from US$ 27 billion in 2010 to US$ 47 billion in 2030 [65].

5. WHAT IS KNOWN ABOUT THE DIRECT COSTS OF STROKE?

Direct costs refer to medical costs associated with diagnosis, treatment and care and non-medical costs such as the cost of transport to a health provider. Many studies have found high direct costs associated with stroke. Direct costs include costs for inpatient stays, outpatient visits, rehabilitation, medications, and nursing home services. Reported health-care costs associated with stroke vary across countries and regions, and across the subtype of stroke. Reported annual direct costs were the highest in the WHO Region of the Americas, followed by the European Region and the Western Pacific Region. The minimum and maximum mean reported annual total direct costs for stroke and heart disease were US$ 6668 [66] and US$ 81 096 [67] in the Region of the Americas, US$ 1643 [68] and US$ 69 440 [69] in the European Region and US$ 3862 [70] and US$ 5693 [71] in the Western Pacific Region, respectively. Worldwide, of all major NCDs, stroke, heart disease and cancer had the highest reported mean annual total direct costs. Hospital costs represent the main driver of stroke expenditure, accounting for 90% [72] of total direct costs. For example, total annual direct costs for stroke alone were estimated at US$ 22.8 billion in 2009 for the United States [73] and €26.6 billion in 2010 for the European Union plus Iceland, Norway and Switzerland [74].

There is limited information available from low- and middle-income countries regarding the cost of stroke treatment. Available data are mostly from retrospective studies conducted in the private health sector. The mean direct medical cost of stroke ranges from US$ 416 in Senegal to US$ 8424 in Nigeria [75]. Length of hospital stay and severity of stroke appear to be the main determinants of hospital costs. Costs of stroke are variable because of the diversity of health-care systems prevailing in low- and middle-income countries [75].

6. HOW DO STROKE COSTS IMPACT ON NATIONAL HEALTH EXPENDITURE?

Some studies conducted in high-income countries have analysed stroke-related long-term costs for survivors and stroke costs as a percentage of national health-care expenditure [56, 61, 63, 76 - 88]. A study in Spain reported the average cost for each stroke survivor at €17 618 in the first year, €14 453 in the second year and €12 924 in the third year after the stroke; the reference year for unit prices was 2004 [56]. In an Australian study the average annual resource use after 12 months was AU$ 6022 for first-ever ischaemic stroke and AU$ 3977 for first-ever haemorrhagic stroke [61]. The average lifetime costs per first-ever ischaemic stroke was AU$ 57 106 and AU$ 49 995 for haemorrhagic stroke [61]. The total costs in the first year accounted for 38% of ischaemic stroke and 53% of haemorrhagic stroke lifetime costs, indicating that haemorrhagic stroke cases are more expensive to treat in the first year. Inpatient hospital costs accounted for about 43% of total costs in the first year for both types of stroke. In the first year, haemorrhagic stroke cases were more expensive to treat than ischaemic stroke in terms of hospitalization, rehabilitation, aged care and use of community services. In contrast, ischaemic stroke cases incurred greater costs for hospitalizations attributable to recurrent events or complications from stroke, caregiver costs, medications and general practitioner care. In this study the total lifetime cost burden of first-ever stroke was estimated at more than AU$ 2 billion in 2004 [61]. A study conducted in the United Kingdom estimated the cost of stroke from a societal perspective, using data from a South London Stroke Register and a number of other national sources [76]. Total societal cost estimates were £8.9 billion per year, with treatment costs accounting for approximately 5% of total United Kingdom National Health Service costs. Direct care accounted for approximately 50% of the total, informal care costs 27% and indirect costs 24%. The breakdown for other cost categories were, approximately, inpatient care 10%, outpatient care 7%, community care 32%, productivity loss 15% and benefit payments 9%. Total annual direct cost of stroke was approximately £4 billion (5.5% of the total United Kingdom expenditure on health care) [76]. From an international perspective, Evers *et al.* reported the percentage of health-care expenditures arising from stroke in six developed countries at 3% on average [77]. Other estimates suggested that stroke consumed more than this average with total direct health-care expenditure on stroke falling between 4% and 6% of National Health Service expenditure [78 - 88].

In the United States in 2005, the annual spending for stroke was US$ 26.8 billion, which was 2% of national health spending [89]. The national cost in the United States increased 7% for subarachnoid haemorrhage, 10% for intracerebral haemorrhage and 18% for acute ischaemic stroke from 2003–2004 to 2011–2012 [90]. Median state costs attributable to stroke were estimated at US$ 873 million (2010 US dollars) (range US$ 86–5959). Across states, Medicaid and Medicare medical costs represented 50.9% of overall state medical costs for stroke [91].

In Canada, a 1-year prospective study was conducted with a cohort of ischaemic stroke patients recruited at 12 Canadian stroke centres to estimate the economic burden of ischaemic stroke [92]. The average annual cost was US$ 74 353; with US$ 107 883 for disabling strokes and US$ 48 339 for non-disabling strokes. Costs during the hospitalization to the 3-months phase were the highest contributor to the annual cost. A rough calculation using 38 000 stroke admissions per year and the average annual cost yielded US$ 2.8 billion as the burden of ischaemic stroke in Canada. In a study conducted in China, expenses associated with hospitalization for cardiovascular diseases increased from 2008 to 2012, constituting 0.16% of national health expenditure in 2012. The total health expenditures for cardiovascular disease was predicted to increase to over US$ 1.71 billion in 2030, if there are no additional government interventions. About two thirds of hospitalization expenditures for cardiovascular disease was from stroke and ischaemic heart disease [93]. Overall, health-care costs due to stroke increased with the severity of the disease, years lived with the condition and co-morbidity [94 - 96].

7. WHAT IS THE COST OF TREATING AN ACUTE STROKE?

Various reviews evaluating patient-level costs of acute stroke care have reported significant variation in cost estimates [82]. In a recent review of 32 studies, direct medical costs were abstracted from the studies for inpatient hospitalization for acute event and follow-up through the first year after an initial event. The mean cost of an acute ischaemic stroke was US$ 18 543 in the United States and US$ 11 900 in Europe [97]. Across all studies, the average cost of an acute ischaemic stroke hospitalization was US$ 11 635 (median: US$ 8097). Costs in the United States ranged from US$ 8069 in a Medicare claims analysis [98] to US$ 38 231 in young patients (aged 18–44) [99]. Acute stroke cost was US$ 13 469 for patients with diabetes [100] and US$ 20 303 for patients with a previous stroke or transient ischaemic attack [101]. The average cost of acute ischaemic stroke across Europe was US$ 11 900, with a low estimate of US$ 5016 in a German hospital cohort [102] and a high estimate of US$ 24 451 in a Scottish population registry [103].

According to a study conducted in China, on average, the overall hospital cost for stroke was US$ 1602, which equates to US$ 81 per day based on an average length of stay of 20 days [104]. Given national average annual wages of US$ 3000 in 2006 [105], this health-care cost translates into more than half a year's wages for many people in China. The total direct costs of stroke in rural South Africa were estimated to be R2.5–4.2 million (US$ 283 500–485 000) in 2012 or 1.6–3% of the subdistrict health expenditure. Out of this, 80% was attributed to inpatient costs [106].

Lower hospital costs for ischaemic stroke than haemorrhagic stroke have been reported from Australia [61] China [104], Greece [107], Japan [108] and the United States [109].

Variations in the hospital costs of acute stroke tend to be determined by stroke severity and length of hospital stay, with patients with more severe neurological impairment on admission requiring assisted feeding, being more disabled at discharge and having longer length of stay, and thus more likely to incur higher costs of care. Other factors associated with increased hospital cost of acute stroke in various studies include having health insurance, higher household income, stroke due to large artery cerebral infarction, greater initial stroke severity, need for assisted feeding, presence of in-hospital complications, long length of stay, being disabled/dependent on discharge and being treated in a tertiary care hospitals in affluent provinces. Higher costs in tertiary care may be indicative of higher probability of severe patients being managed in larger referral hospitals, and higher staff, infrastructure costs and overheads for hospitals in more affluent provinces.

8. WHAT IS THE COST OF ATRIAL FIBRILLATION-RELATED STROKE?

Atrial fibrillation is the most common cardiac arrhythmia and occurs most commonly in older populations. It is a well-recognized risk factor for ischaemic stroke and transient ischaemic attacks. There is a 2-fold to 3.5-fold increase in the risk of stroke among those with atrial fibrillation when compared to those without it [110]. As discussed in chapter 1, approximately 15–20% of patients experiencing ischaemic stroke have atrial fibrillation [111, 112]. Stroke severity and in-hospital mortality are also significantly greater in those with atrial fibrillation [111, 112]. Increased life expectancy in both developed and developing countries means that atrial fibrillation-related stroke has become a growing global public health issue.

Several studies have reported the excess cost of atrial fibrillation-related stroke compared with non-atrial fibrillation-related stroke [113 - 115]. In all of the studies, the direct costs of stroke were greater in patients with atrial fibrillation than in those without it. Atrial fibrillation-related stroke costs an average of between 7% and 20% more than non-atrial fibrillation-related stroke [113 - 115]. The excess cost was attributable to higher acute care costs, longer lengths of hospital stay and greater frequency of recurrent stroke events over a 3-year period [114]. The total lifetime costs of atrial fibrillation-related strokes occurring in a single year were estimated in an Australian report at AU\$ 215.7 million in 2008–2009 [116].

9. WHAT ARE THE HOSPITAL COSTS OF STROKE BASED ON POPULATION STUDIES?

Long-term hospital costs after stroke are increasing with prolonged survival and the ageing population. To reliably determine the long-term hospital costs after stroke, population-based studies with full case ascertainment are required. Case ascertainment needs to include minor events not admitted to the hospital and strokes resulting in death before, or soon after, hospital admission. There are few such studies from high-income countries [43, 55, 117].

In a population-based study conducted in Australia, the total average lifetime cost per case was estimated at AU\$ 64 733 for ischaemic stroke and AU\$ 54 721 for haemorrhagic stroke [55]. The total lifetime costs for all first-ever ischaemic and haemorrhagic stroke events in 2004 was approximately AU\$ 2 billion. Total outpatient and community costs were greater than costs of inpatient hospital care for both ischaemic and haemorrhagic stroke. The total costs in the first year accounted for 38% of ischaemic stroke and 53% of haemorrhagic stroke lifetime costs. Inpatient hospital costs accounted for about 43% of total costs in the first year for both types of stroke. In the first year, haemorrhagic stroke cases were more expensive to treat than ischaemic stroke in terms of hospitalization, rehabilitation, aged care and use of community services. Greater costs were incurred for ischaemic stroke cases for hospitalizations attributable to recurrent events or complications from stroke, caregiver costs, medications, general practitioner care and investigations.

Another population-based study estimated costs from individual patient data at the national level in Finland [115]. For patients in 2007, the mean 1-year costs after an ischaemic stroke were US$ 29 580, after an intracerebral haemorrhage US$ 36 220 and after a subarachnoid haemorrhage US$ 42 570, valued in 2008 US dollars. The annual costs prior to stroke were US$ 8900 before ischaemic stroke, US$ 7600 before intracerebral haemorrhage and US$ 4200 before subarachnoid haemorrhage. Older patients with ischaemic stroke and, among patients with ischaemic stroke and subarachnoid haemorrhage, women incurred higher costs. The mean estimated lifetime costs were US$ 130 000 after ischaemic stroke or intracerebral haemorrhage and US$ 80 000 after subarachnoid haemorrhage. Annually, US$ 1.6 billion is spent in the care of Finnish patients with stroke, which equals to 7% of the national health-care expenditure, or 0.6% of GDP.

In a more recent population-based cohort study conducted in the United Kingdom, 5-year hospital costs after index stroke were US$ 25 741, with costs varying considerably by severity: US$ 21 134 after minor stroke, US$ 33 119 after moderate stroke and US$ 28 552 after severe stroke [117]. For surviving stroke patients who reached final follow-up, mean costs were US$ 24 383, with over half of costs being incurred in the first year after the event. After index transient ischaemic attacks, the mean 5-year costs were US$ 18 091 (US$ 15 947–20 258). Event severity, recurrent stroke and coronary events after the index event were independent predictors of 5-year costs.

10. WHAT ARE THE SOCIAL COSTS AND CONSEQUENCES OF STROKE?

A systematic review has examined social consequences of stroke for working-age people [43]. Categories of social consequences of stroke included negative impact on family relationships (5–54%) [118 - 121], deterioration of sexual life (5–76%) [119 - 122, 124], economic difficulties (24–33%) [119, 122, 123, 125] and deterioration in leisure activities (15–79%) [118, 124, 126]. Marital problems after stroke have been reported, including conflict with spouse, deterioration in the spousal relationship, separation and divorce [120, 123, 125, 126]. Effects of stroke for children include parent–child conflict, difficulties with child care and impact on children as caregivers [119 - 121, 123].

Studies showed that stroke patients already exert a significant burden on health and social welfare systems even before their stroke. Patients and their partners have high rates of contact with all sectors of the health-care system. This covers contact with general practice, outpatient clinics and in-hospital services, as well as medication use, and publicly supported payment for medication. Health-care contacts are more frequent in the secondary health-care system, in which partners make greater demands on the social care system, and consequently incur greater direct and indirect costs [127]. Social and health costs also increase over time for caregivers of stroke victims [56]

11. WHAT ARE THE ECONOMIC CONSEQUENCES OF STROKE ON HOUSEHOLDS?

Stroke (NCDs) pose a heavy financial burden on affected households. Limited insurance coverage and lack of social security nets force households to spend large amounts of money on out-of-pocket expenses. Low-income households are especially vulnerable to impoverishment from health-care spending due to NCDs.

Household income losses after diagnosis of heart disease and stroke were 14.3%, 26.3%, 63.5% and 67.5% in high-income families in China, India, the United Republic of Tanzania and Argentina, respectively, and were even higher in the lower-income groups [128].

With regard to stroke, the average out-of-pocket burden as a percentage of income in Japan ranged between 5.1 and 17.2% [129]. In China, out-of-pocket costs in the first three months after diagnosis of stroke was 158% greater than the annual income. Catastrophic spending (*e.g.* out-of-pocket spending as 30% of annual income) was experienced by 71% of patients, pushing an estimated 23% of insured and 62% of uninsured stroke patients below the US$ 1 per day poverty line [130]. In the United States, 27.8% of stroke patients reported out-of-pocket spending at 20% of the family income [131]. Among Australian stroke survivors, an estimated US$ 473 was spent in the first year after diagnosis and 61% experienced financial hardship after 12 months [132, 133].

Out-of-pocket payments for the treatment of stroke lead to significant costs for households. Up to 71% of patients who had experienced an acute stroke faced catastrophic health expenditure in China, while 37% of them fell below the poverty line of US$ 1 per day after paying for their health care [130]. Catastrophic payments and impoverishment due to stroke was more common in people with no health insurance than in those with health insurance [130]. Other factors that predicted catastrophic payments were being the main income earner in the household, a manual worker, lower level of education, having an intracerebral haemorrhage, a severe stroke at admission, being disabled at hospital discharge and having multiple readmissions to the hospital [130].

CONCLUDING REMARKS

There are considerable differences in costs from productivity loss due to stroke between countries. There is also likely to be a differential impact of stroke on economic productivity in high-income and low- and middle- income countries because case fatality and disability rates are higher in low- and middle-income countries compared to high-income countries. The impact that stroke exerts on households and impoverishment is likely to be underestimated as important economic areas such as coping strategies and the inclusion of vulnerable segments of the population who do not seek health care due to health system limitations are overlooked in published studies. Future research to estimate the economic impact of stroke needs to rectify the scarcity of reliable country-specific information on stroke for many low- and middle-income countries. These data are essential to make a convincing case to Governments, to invest more in prevention and control of stroke.

CONFLICT OF INTEREST

The author declares no conflict of interest, financial or otherwise.

ACKNOWLEDGEMENTS

Ms AvisAnne Julien is thanked for copy-editing.

REFERENCES

[1]   Global status report on noncommunicable diseases 2014 Attaining the nine global NCD targets: a shared responsibility. Geneva: World Health Organization 2014.

[2]   WHO Guide to identifying the economic impact of disease and injury. Geneva: World Health Organization 2009.

[3]   Chaker L, Falla A, van der Lee SJ, *et al.* The global impact of non-communicable diseases on macro-economic productivity: a systematic review. Eur J Epidemiol 2015; 30(5): 357-95.
       [http://dx.doi.org/10.1007/s10654-015-0026-5] [PMID: 25837965]

[4]   Jaspers L, Colpani V, Chaker L, *et al.* The global impact of non-communicable diseases on households and impoverishment: a systematic review. Eur J Epidemiol 2015; 30(3): 163-88.
       [http://dx.doi.org/10.1007/s10654-014-9983-3] [PMID: 25527371]

[5]   Muka T, Imo D, Jaspers L, *et al.* The global impact of non-communicable diseases on healthcare spending and national income: a systematic review. Eur J Epidemiol 2015; 30(4): 251-77.
       [http://dx.doi.org/10.1007/s10654-014-9984-2] [PMID: 25595318]

[6]   Bloom DE, Cafiero ET, Jané-Llopis E, Abrahams-Gessel S, Bloom LR, Fathima S, *et al.* The global economic burden of noncommunicable diseases. Geneva: World Economic Forum.

[7]   From burden to "best buys": reducing the economic impact of NCDs in low- and middle-income countries/ Geneva: WHO and World Economic Forum 2011. Available at: http://www.who.int/ nmh/publications/best_buys_summary/en/

[8]   Global action plan for the prevention and control of noncommunicable diseases 2013-2020. 2013. Available at: http://apps.who.int/iris/bitstream/10665/94384/1/9789241506236_ eng.pdf?ua=1

[9]   Scaling up action against noncommunicable diseases: How much will it cost?. Geneva, Switzerland: World Health Organization 2011.

[10]   Gènova-Maleras R, Álvarez-Martín E, Morant-Ginestar C, Fernández de Larrea-Baz N, Catalá-López F. Measuring the burden of disease and injury in Spain using disability-adjusted life years: an updated and policy-oriented overview. Public Health 2012; 126(12): 1024-31.
[http://dx.doi.org/10.1016/j.puhe.2012.08.012] [PMID: 23062632]

[11]   Catala-Lopez F, Fernandez de Larrea-Baz N, Morant-Ginestar C, Alvarez-Martin E, Diaz-Guzman J, Genova-Maleras R. The national burden of cerebrovascular diseases in Spain: a population-based study using disability-adjusted life years. Med Clin (Barc) 2014; •••
[http://dx.doi.org/10.1016/j.medcli.2013.11.040] [PMID: 24863563]

[12]   Katzenellenbogen JM, Vos T, Somerford P, Begg S, Semmens JB, Codde JP. Burden of stroke in indigenous Western Australians: a study using data linkage. Stroke 2011; 42(6): 1515-21.
[http://dx.doi.org/10.1161/STROKEAHA.110.601799] [PMID: 21493909]

[13]   Modrego PJ, Mainar R, Turull L. Recurrence and survival after first-ever stroke in the area of Bajo Aragon, Spain. A prospective cohort study. J Neurol Sci 2004; 224(1-2): 49-55.
[http://dx.doi.org/10.1016/j.jns.2004.06.002] [PMID: 15450771]

[14]   Arrazola A, Beguiristain JM, Garitano B, Mar J, Elizalde B. Atención hospitalaria a la enfermedad cerebrovascular aguda y situación de los pacientes a los 12 meses. Rev Neurol 2005; 40(6): 326-30.
[PMID: 15795867]

[15]   Jørgensen HS, Kammersgaard LP, Nakayama H, *et al.* Treatment and rehabilitation on a stroke unit improves 5-year survival. A community-based study. Stroke 1999; 30(5): 930-3.
[http://dx.doi.org/10.1161/01.STR.30.5.930] [PMID: 10229722]

[16]   Kang HY, Lim SJ, Suh HS, Liew D. Estimating the lifetime economic burden of stroke according to the age of onset in South Korea: a cost of illness study. BMC Public Health 2011; 11: 646.
[http://dx.doi.org/10.1186/1471-2458-11-646] [PMID: 21838919]

[17]   Kabadi GS, Walker R, Donaldson C, Shackley P. The cost of treating stroke in urban and rural Tanzania: a 6-month pilot study. Afr J Neurol Sci 2013; 32(2)

[18]   Gabriele W, Renate S. Work loss following stroke. Disabil Rehabil 2009; 31(18): 1487-93.
[http://dx.doi.org/10.1080/09638280802621432] [PMID: 19479493]

[19]   Hackett ML, Glozier N, Jan S, Lindley R. Returning to paid employment after stroke: the Psychosocial Outcomes in Stroke (POISE) cohort study. PLoS ONE 2012.

[20]   Quinn AC, Bhargava D, Al-Tamimi YZ, Clark MJ, Ross SA, Tennant A. Self-perceived health status following aneurysmal subarachnoid haemorrhage: a cohort study. BMJ Open 2014; 4(4): e003932.
[http://dx.doi.org/10.1136/bmjopen-2013-003932] [PMID: 24699459]

[21]   Korea center for disease control and prevention. The Korea national health and nutrition examination survey (KNHANES I). Seoul: Korea Ministry of Health, Welfare, and Family Affairs 1998.

[22]   Korea center for disease control and prevention. The Korea national health and nutrition examination survey (KNHANES III). Seoul: Korea Ministry of Health, Welfare, and Family Affairs 2005.

[23]   Kim AS, Johnston SC. Global variation in the relative burden of stroke and ischemic heart disease. Circulation 2011; 124(3): 314-23.
[http://dx.doi.org/10.1161/CIRCULATIONAHA.111.018820] [PMID: 21730306]

[24]   Yusuf S, Reddy S, Ounpuu S, Anand S. Global burden of cardiovascular diseases: part I: general considerations, the epidemiologic transition, risk factors, and impact of urbanization. Circulation 2001; 104(22): 2746-53.
[http://dx.doi.org/10.1161/hc4601.099487] [PMID: 11723030]

[25]   Luengo-Fernandez R, Gray AM, Rothwell PM. Costs of stroke using patient-level data: a critical review of the literature. Stroke 2009; 40(2): e18-23.

[http://dx.doi.org/10.1161/STROKEAHA.108.529776] [PMID: 19109540]

[26]   Feigin VL. Stroke in developing countries: can the epidemic be stopped and outcomes improved? Lancet Neurol 2007; 6(2): 94-7.
[http://dx.doi.org/10.1016/S1474-4422(07)70007-8] [PMID: 17239789]

[27]   Brown DL, Boden-Albala B, Langa KM, *et al.* Projected costs of ischemic stroke in the United States. Neurology 2006; 67(8): 1390-5.
[http://dx.doi.org/10.1212/01.wnl.0000237024.16438.20] [PMID: 16914694]

[28]   Tanaka H, Toyonaga T, Hashimoto H. Functional and occupational characteristics associated with very early return to work after stroke in Japan. Arch Phys Med Rehabil 2011; 92(5): 743-8.
[http://dx.doi.org/10.1016/j.apmr.2010.12.009] [PMID: 21530721]

[29]   Saeki S. Disability management after stroke: its medical aspects for workplace accommodation. Disabil Rehabil 2000; 22(13-14): 578-82.
[http://dx.doi.org/10.1080/09638280050138241] [PMID: 11052206]

[30]   Singhal AB, Lo W. Life after stroke: Beyond medications. Neurology 2014; 83(13): 1128-9.
[http://dx.doi.org/10.1212/WNL.0000000000000827] [PMID: 25128181]

[31]   Palmer AJ, Valentine WJ, Roze S, Lammert M, Spiesser J, Gabriel S. Overview of costs of stroke from published, incidence-based studies spanning 16 industrialized countries. Curr Med Res Opin 2005; 21(1): 19-26.
[http://dx.doi.org/10.1185/030079904X17992] [PMID: 15881472]

[32]   Kisoli A, Gray WK, Dotchin CL, *et al.* Levels of functional disability in elderly people in Tanzania with dementia, stroke and Parkinson's disease. Acta Neuropsychiatr 2015; 27(4): 206-12.
[http://dx.doi.org/10.1017/neu.2015.9] [PMID: 25777617]

[33]   Ekenze OS, Onwuekwe IO, Ezeala Adikaibe BA. Profile of neurological admissions at the University of Nigeria Teaching Hospital Enugu. Niger J Med 2010; 19(4): 419-22.
[http://dx.doi.org/10.4314/njm.v19i4.61967] [PMID: 21526631]

[34]   Walker R, Whiting D, Unwin N, *et al.* Stroke incidence in rural and urban Tanzania: a prospective, community-based study. Lancet Neurol 2010; 9(8): 786-92.
[http://dx.doi.org/10.1016/S1474-4422(10)70144-7] [PMID: 20609629]

[35]   Walker RW, Jusabani A, Aris E, *et al.* Post-stroke case fatality within an incident population in rural Tanzania. J Neurol Neurosurg Psychiatry 2011; 82(9): 1001-5.
[http://dx.doi.org/10.1136/jnnp.2010.231944] [PMID: 21386108]

[36]   O'Donnell MJ, Xavier D, Liu L, *et al.* Risk factors for ischaemic and intracerebral haemorrhagic stroke in 22 countries (the INTERSTROKE study): a case-control study. Lancet 2010; 376(9735): 112-23.
[http://dx.doi.org/10.1016/S0140-6736(10)60834-3] [PMID: 20561675]

[37]   Endo M, Sairenchi T, Kojimahara N, *et al.* Sickness absence and return to work among Japanese stroke survivors: a 365-day cohort study. BMJ Open 2016; 6(1): e009682.
[http://dx.doi.org/10.1136/bmjopen-2015-009682] [PMID: 26729388]

[38]   Saeki S, Toyonaga T. Determinants of early return to work after first stroke in Japan. J Rehabil Med 2010; 42(3): 254-8.
[http://dx.doi.org/10.2340/16501977-0503] [PMID: 20411221]

[39]   Glozier N, Hackett ML, Parag V, Anderson CS. The influence of psychiatric morbidity on return to paid work after stroke in younger adults: the Auckland Regional Community Stroke (ARCOS) Study, 2002 to 2003. Stroke 2008; 39(5): 1526-32.
[http://dx.doi.org/10.1161/STROKEAHA.107.503219] [PMID: 18369172]

[40]   Saeki S, Ogata H, Okubo T, Takahashi K, Hoshuyama T. Factors influencing return to work after stroke in Japan. Stroke 1993; 24(8): 1182-5.
[http://dx.doi.org/10.1161/01.STR.24.8.1182] [PMID: 8342194]

[41] Busch MA, Coshall C, Heuschmann PU, McKevitt C, Wolfe CD. Sociodemographic differences in return to work after stroke: the South London Stroke Register (SLSR). J Neurol Neurosurg Psychiatry 2009; 80(8): 888-93.
[http://dx.doi.org/10.1136/jnnp.2008.163295] [PMID: 19276102]

[42] Hannerz H, Mortensen OS, Poulsen OM, Humle F, Pedersen BH, Andersen LL. Time trend analysis of return to work after stroke in Denmark 1996-2006. Int J Occup Med Environ Health 2012; 25(2): 200-4.
[http://dx.doi.org/10.2478/s13382-012-0017-7] [PMID: 22492285]

[43] Daniel K, Wolfe CD, Busch MA, McKevitt C. What are the social consequences of stroke for working-aged adults? A systematic review. Stroke 2009; 40(6): e431-40.
[http://dx.doi.org/10.1161/STROKEAHA.108.534487] [PMID: 19390074]

[44] Gilworth G, Phil M, Cert A, Sansam KA, Kent RM. Personal experiences of returning to work following stroke: An exploratory study. Work 2009; 34(1): 95-103.
[PMID: 19923680]

[45] Saeki S, Hachisuka K. The association between stroke location and return to work after first stroke. J Stroke Cerebrovasc Dis 2004; 13(4): 160-3.
[http://dx.doi.org/10.1016/j.jstrokecerebrovasdis.2004.06.006] [PMID: 17903969]

[46] Hannerz H, Pedersen BH, Poulsen OM, Humle F, Andersen LL. Study protocol to a nationwide prospective cohort study on return to gainful occupation after stroke in Denmark 1996 - 2006. BMC Public Health 2010; 10: 623.
[http://dx.doi.org/10.1186/1471-2458-10-623] [PMID: 20958997]

[47] Hannerz H, Holbæk Pedersen B, Poulsen OM, Humle F, Andersen LL. A nationwide prospective cohort study on return to gainful occupation after stroke in Denmark 1996-2006. BMJ Open 2011; 1(2): e000180.
[http://dx.doi.org/10.1136/bmjopen-2011-000180] [PMID: 22021879]

[48] Ganapathy V, Graham GD, DiBonaventura MD, Gillard PJ, Goren A, Zorowitz RD. Caregiver burden, productivity loss, and indirect costs associated with caring for patients with poststroke spasticity. Clin Interv Aging 2015; 10: 1793-802.
[PMID: 26609225]

[49] Zheng H, Ehrlich F, Amin J. Productivity loss resulting from coronary heart disease in Australia. Appl Health Econ Health Policy 2010; 8(3): 179-89.
[http://dx.doi.org/10.2165/11530520-000000000-00000] [PMID: 20408602]

[50] van den Berg B, Brouwer W, van Exel J, Koopmanschap M, van den Bos GA, Rutten F. Economic valuation of informal care: lessons from the application of the opportunity costs and proxy good methods. Soc Sci Med 2006; 62(4): 835-45.
[http://dx.doi.org/10.1016/j.socscimed.2005.06.046] [PMID: 16137814]

[51] Joo H, George MG, Fang J, Wang G. A literature review of indirect costs associated with stroke. J Stroke Cerebrovasc Dis 2014; 23(7): 1753-63.
[http://dx.doi.org/10.1016/j.jstrokecerebrovasdis.2014.02.017] [PMID: 24957313]

[52] Rossnagel K, Nolte CH, Muller-Nordhorn J, *et al.* Medical resource use and costs of health care after acute stroke in Germany. Eur J Neurol 2005; 12(11): 862-8.
[http://dx.doi.org/10.1111/j.1468-1331.2005.01091.x] [PMID: 16241975]

[53] Ghatnekar O, Persson U, Glader EL, Terént A. Cost of stroke in Sweden: an incidence estimate. Int J Technol Assess Health Care 2004; 20(3): 375-80.
[http://dx.doi.org/10.1017/S0266462304001217] [PMID: 15446769]

[54] Navarrete-Navarro P, Hart WM, Lopez-Bastida J, Christensen MC. The societal costs of intracerebral hemorrhage in Spain. Eur J Neurol 2007; 14(5): 556-62.
[http://dx.doi.org/10.1111/j.1468-1331.2007.01756.x] [PMID: 17437616]

[55]   Cadilhac DA, Carter R, Thrift AG, Dewey HM. Estimating the long-term costs of ischemic and hemorrhagic stroke for Australia: new evidence derived from the North East Melbourne Stroke Incidence Study (NEMESIS). Stroke 2009; 40(3): 915-21.
[http://dx.doi.org/10.1161/STROKEAHA.108.526905] [PMID: 19182091]

[56]   Lopez-Bastida J, Oliva Moreno J, Worbes Cerezo M, Perestelo Perez L, Serrano-Aguilar P, Montón-Álvarez F. Social and economic costs and health-related quality of life in stroke survivors in the Canary Islands, Spain. BMC Health Serv Res 2012; 12: 315.
[http://dx.doi.org/10.1186/1472-6963-12-315] [PMID: 22970797]

[57]   Wiebers DO, Torner JC, Meissner I. Impact of unruptured intracranial aneurysms on public health in the United States. Stroke 1992; 23(10): 1416-9.
[http://dx.doi.org/10.1161/01.STR.23.10.1416] [PMID: 1412577]

[58]   Riewpaiboon A, Riewpaiboon W, Ponsoongnern K, Van den Berg B. Economic valuation of informal care in Asia: a case study of care for disabled stroke survivors in Thailand. Soc Sci Med 2009; 69(4): 648-53.
[http://dx.doi.org/10.1016/j.socscimed.2009.05.033] [PMID: 19573969]

[59]   Persson J, Ferraz-Nunes J, Karlberg I. Economic burden of stroke in a large county in Sweden. BMC Health Serv Res 2012; 12: 341.
[http://dx.doi.org/10.1186/1472-6963-12-341] [PMID: 23013284]

[60]   Terént A, Marké LA, Asplund K, Norrving B, Jonsson E, Wester PO. Costs of stroke in Sweden. A national perspective. Stroke 1994; 25(12): 2363-9.
[http://dx.doi.org/10.1161/01.STR.25.12.2363] [PMID: 7974574]

[61]   Dewey HM, Thrift AG, Mihalopoulos C, *et al.* Cost of stroke in Australia from a societal perspective: results from the North East Melbourne Stroke Incidence Study (NEMESIS). Stroke 2001; 32(10): 2409-16.
[http://dx.doi.org/10.1161/hs1001.097222] [PMID: 11588334]

[62]   Scott WG, Scott H. Ischaemic stroke in New Zealand: an economic study. N Z Med J 1994; 107(989): 443-6.
[PMID: 7970352]

[63]   Hickenbottom SL, Fendrick AM, Kutcher JS, Kabeto MU, Katz SJ, Langa KM. A national study of the quantity and cost of informal caregiving for the elderly with stroke. Neurology 2002; 58(12): 1754-9.
[http://dx.doi.org/10.1212/WNL.58.12.1754] [PMID: 12084872]

[64]   Fox P, Gazzaniga J, Karter A, Max W. The economic costs of cardiovascular disease mortality in California, 1991: implications for public health policy. J Public Health Policy 1996; 17(4): 442-59.
[http://dx.doi.org/10.2307/3343102] [PMID: 9009539]

[65]   Heidenreich PA, Trogdon JG, Khavjou OA, *et al.* American Heart Association Advocacy Coordinating Committee; Stroke Council; Council on Cardiovascular Radiology and Intervention; Council on Clinical Cardiology; Council on Epidemiology and Prevention; Council on Arteriosclerosis; Thrombosis and Vascular Biology; Council on Cardiopulmonary; Critical Care; Perioperative and Resuscitation; Council on Cardiovascular Nursing; Council on the Kidney in Cardiovascular Disease; Council on Cardiovascular Surgery and Anesthesia, and Interdisciplinary Council on Quality of Care and Outcomes Research. Forecasting the future of cardiovascular disease in the United States: a policy statement from the American Heart Association. Circulation 2011; 123(8): 933-44.
[http://dx.doi.org/10.1161/CIR.0b013e31820a55f5] [PMID: 21262990]

[66]   Anis AH, Guh D, Stieb D, *et al.* The costs of cardiorespiratory disease episodes in a study of emergency department use. Can J Public Health 2000; 91(2): 103-6.
[PMID: 10832172]

[67]   Unroe KT, Greiner MA, Hernandez AF, *et al.* Resource use in the last 6 months of life among medicare beneficiaries with heart failure, 2000-2007. Arch Intern Med 2011; 171(3): 196-203.
        [http://dx.doi.org/10.1001/archinternmed.2010.371] [PMID: 20937916]

[68]   Jaworski R, Jankowska EA, Ponikowski P, Banasiak W. Costs of management of patients with coronary artery disease in Poland: the multicenter RECENT study. Pol Arch Med Wewn 2012; 122(12): 599-607.
        [http://dx.doi.org/10.20452/pamw.1533] [PMID: 23160000]

[69]   Ward A, Payne KA, Caro JJ, Heuschmann PU, Kolominsky-Rabas PL. Care needs and economic consequences after acute ischemic stroke: the Erlangen Stroke Project. Eur J Neurol 2005; 12(4): 264-7.
        [http://dx.doi.org/10.1111/j.1468-1331.2004.00949.x] [PMID: 15804242]

[70]   Ademi Z, Liew D, Zomer E, *et al.* Outcomes and excess costs among patients with cardiovascular disease. Heart Lung Circ 2013; 22(9): 724-30.
        [http://dx.doi.org/10.1016/j.hlc.2013.02.002] [PMID: 23510668]

[71]   Lee HC, Chang KC, Huang YC, *et al.* Readmission, mortality, and first-year medical costs after stroke. J Chin Med Assoc 2013; 76(12): 703-14.
        [http://dx.doi.org/10.1016/j.jcma.2013.08.003] [PMID: 24075791]

[72]   Bottacchi E, Corso G, Tosi P, *et al.* The cost of first-ever stroke in Valle d'Aosta, Italy: linking clinical registries and administrative data. BMC Health Serv Res 2012; 12: 372.
        [http://dx.doi.org/10.1186/1472-6963-12-372] [PMID: 23110322]

[73]   Go AS, Mozaffarian D, Roger VL, *et al.* American Heart Association Statistics Committee and Stroke Statistics Subcommittee. Heart disease and stroke statistics--2013 update: a report from the American Heart Association. Circulation 2013; 127(1): e6-e245.
        [http://dx.doi.org/10.1161/CIR.0b013e31828124ad] [PMID: 23239837]

[74]   Gustavsson A, Svensson M, Jacobi F, *et al.* CDBE2010Study Group. Cost of disorders of the brain in Europe 2010. Eur Neuropsychopharmacol 2011; 21(10): 718-79.
        [http://dx.doi.org/10.1016/j.euroneuro.2011.08.008] [PMID: 21924589]

[75]   Kaur P1, Kwatra G, Kaur R, Pandian JD. Cost of stroke in low- and middle-income countries: a systematic review. Int J Stroke Augist 2014; 9(6): 678-82. [Epub 7 July 2014].
        [http://dx.doi.org/10.1111/ijs.12322]

[76]   Saka O, McGuire A, Wolfe C. Cost of stroke in the United Kingdom. Age Ageing 2009; 38(1): 27-32.
        [http://dx.doi.org/10.1093/ageing/afn281] [PMID: 19141506]

[77]   Evers SM, Struijs JN, Ament AJ, van Genugten ML, Jager JH, van den Bos GA. International comparison of stroke cost studies. Stroke 2004; 35(5): 1209-15.
        [http://dx.doi.org/10.1161/01.STR.0000125860.48180.48] [PMID: 15073405]

[78]   Stegmayr B, Asplund K. Stroke in Northern Sweden. Scand J Public Health Suppl 2003; 61: 60-9.
        [http://dx.doi.org/10.1080/14034950310001379] [PMID: 14660249]

[79]   Taylor TN, Davis PH, Torner JC, Holmes J, Meyer JW, Jacobson MF. Lifetime cost of stroke in the United States. Stroke 1996; 27(9): 1459-66.
        [http://dx.doi.org/10.1161/01.STR.27.9.1459] [PMID: 8784113]

[80]   Persson U, Silverberg R, Lindgren B, *et al.* Direct costs of stroke for a Swedish population. Int J Technol Assess Health Care 1990; 6(1): 125-37.
        [http://dx.doi.org/10.1017/S0266462300008989] [PMID: 2113889]

[81]   Porsdal V, Boysen G. Cost-of illness studies of stroke. Cerebrovasc Dis 1997; 7: 258-63.
        [http://dx.doi.org/10.1159/000108204]

[82]   Payne KA, Huybrechts KF, Caro JJ, Craig Green TJ, Klittich WS. Long term cost-of-illness in stroke: an international review. Pharmacoeconomics 2002; 20(12): 813-25.

[http://dx.doi.org/10.2165/00019053-200220120-00002] [PMID: 12236803]

[83]   Evers SM, Engel GL, Ament AJ. Cost of stroke in The Netherlands from a societal perspective. Stroke 1997; 28(7): 1375-81.
[http://dx.doi.org/10.1161/01.STR.28.7.1375] [PMID: 9227686]

[84]   Beguiristain JM, Mar J, Arrazola A. The cost of cerebrovascular accident. Rev Neurol 2005; 40(7): 406-11.
[PMID: 15849673]

[85]   Weimar C, Weber C, Wagner M, *et al.* German Stroke Data Bank Collaborators. Management patterns and health care use after intracerebral hemorrhage. a cost-of-illness study from a societal perspective in Germany. Cerebrovasc Dis 2003; 15(1-2): 29-36.
[http://dx.doi.org/10.1159/000067119] [PMID: 12499708]

[86]   Luengo-Fernández R, Leal J, Gray A, Petersen S, Rayner M. Cost of cardiovascular diseases in the United Kingdom. Heart 2006; 92(10): 1384-9.
[http://dx.doi.org/10.1136/hrt.2005.072173] [PMID: 16702172]

[87]   Mitchell JB, Ballard DJ, Whisnant JP, Ammering CJ, Samsa GP, Matchar DB. What role do neurologists play in determining the costs and outcomes of stroke patients? Stroke 1996; 27(11): 1937-43.
[http://dx.doi.org/10.1161/01.STR.27.11.1937] [PMID: 8898795]

[88]   Youman P, Wilson K, Harraf F, Kalra L. The economic burden of stroke in the United Kingdom. Pharmacoeconomics 2003; 21 (Suppl. 1): 43-50.
[http://dx.doi.org/10.2165/00019053-200321001-00005] [PMID: 12648034]

[89]   Roehrig C, Miller G, Lake C, Bryant J. National health spending by medical condition, 1996-2005. Health Aff (Millwood) 2009; 28(2): w358-67.
[http://dx.doi.org/10.1377/hlthaff.28.2.w358] [PMID: 19240056]

[90]   Tong X, George MG, Gillespie C, Merritt R. Trends in hospitalizations and cost associated with stroke by age, United States 2003-2012. Int J Stroke 2016; 11(8): 874-81.
[http://dx.doi.org/10.1177/1747493016654490] [PMID: 27312679]

[91]   Trogdon JG, Murphy LB, Khavjou OA, *et al.* Costs of chronic diseases at the state level: the chronic disease cost calculator. Prev Chronic Dis 2015; 12: E140.
[http://dx.doi.org/10.5888/pcd12.150131] [PMID: 26334712]

[92]   Mittmann N, Seung SJ, Hill MD, *et al.* Impact of disability status on ischemic stroke costs in Canada in the first year. Can J Neurol Sci 2012; 39(6): 793-800.
[http://dx.doi.org/10.1017/S0317167100015638] [PMID: 23041400]

[93]   Wang S, Petzold M, Cao J, Zhang Y, Wang W. Direct medical costs of hospitalizations for cardiovascular diseases in Shanghai, China: trends and projections. Medicine (Baltimore) 2015; 94(20): e837.
[http://dx.doi.org/10.1097/MD.0000000000000837] [PMID: 25997060]

[94]   Claesson L, Gosman-Hedström G, Johannesson M, Fagerberg B, Blomstrand C. Resource utilization and costs of stroke unit care integrated in a care continuum: A 1-year controlled, prospective, randomized study in elderly patients: the Göteborg 70+ Stroke Study. Stroke 2000; 31(11): 2569-77.
[http://dx.doi.org/10.1161/01.STR.31.11.2569] [PMID: 11062277]

[95]   Nor Azlin MN, Syed Aljunid SJ, Noor Azahz A, Amrizal MN, Saperi S. Direct medical cost of stroke: findings from a tertiary hospital in Malaysia. Med J Malaysia 2012; 67(5): 473-7.
[PMID: 23770861]

[96]   Dalal AA, Shah M, Lunacsek O, Hanania NA. Clinical and economic burden of patients diagnosed with COPD with comorbid cardiovascular disease. Respir Med 2011; 105(10): 1516-22.
[http://dx.doi.org/10.1016/j.rmed.2011.04.005] [PMID: 21684731]

[97] Nicholson G, Gandra SR, Halbert RJ, Richhariya A, Nordyke RJ. Patient-level costs of major cardiovascular conditions: a review of the international literature. Clinicoecon Outcomes Res 2016; 8: 495-506.
[http://dx.doi.org/10.2147/CEOR.S89331] [PMID: 27703385]

[98] Lee WC, Christensen MC, Joshi AV, Pashos CL. Long-term cost of stroke subtypes among Medicare beneficiaries. Cerebrovasc Dis 2007; 23(1): 57-65.
[http://dx.doi.org/10.1159/000096542] [PMID: 17065788]

[99] Ellis C. Stroke in young adults. Disabil Health J 2010; 3(3): 222-4.
[http://dx.doi.org/10.1016/j.dhjo.2010.01.001] [PMID: 21122787]

[100] Straka RJ, Liu LZ, Girase PS, DeLorenzo A, Chapman RH. Incremental cardiovascular costs and resource use associated with diabetes: an assessment of 29,863 patients in the US managed-care setting. Cardiovasc Diabetol 2009; 8: 53.
[http://dx.doi.org/10.1186/1475-2840-8-53] [PMID: 19781099]

[101] Engel-Nitz NM, Sander SD, Harley C, Rey GG, Shah H. Costs and outcomes of noncardioembolic ischemic stroke in a managed care population. Vasc Health Risk Manag 2010; 6: 905-13.
[http://dx.doi.org/10.2147/VHRM.S10851] [PMID: 20957133]

[102] Winter Y, Wolfram C, Schaeg M, *et al.* Evaluation of costs and outcome in cardioembolic stroke or TIA. J Neurol 2009; 256(6): 954-63.
[http://dx.doi.org/10.1007/s00415-009-5053-2] [PMID: 19252783]

[103] Zorowitz RD, Chen E, Tong KB, Laouri M. Costs and rehabilitation use of stroke survivors: a retrospective study of Medicare beneficiaries. Top Stroke Rehabil 2009; 16(5): 309-20.
[http://dx.doi.org/10.1310/tsr1605-309] [PMID: 19903649]

[104] Wei JW, Heeley EL, Jan S, *et al.* China QUEST Investigators. Variations and determinants of hospital costs for acute stroke in China. PLoS One 2010; 5(9): e13041.
[http://dx.doi.org/10.1371/journal.pone.0013041] [PMID: 20927384]

[105] National Bureau of Statistics of China. Li X, Ed. China Statistical Yearbook 2007. China Statistics Press. 2007.

[106] Maredza M, Chola L. Economic burden of stroke in a rural South African setting. eNeurological Sci 2016; 3: 26-32.

[107] Gioldasis G, Talelli P, Chroni E, Daouli J, Papapetropoulos T, Ellul J. In-hospital direct cost of acute ischemic and hemorrhagic stroke in Greece. Acta Neurol Scand 2008; 118(4): 268-74.
[http://dx.doi.org/10.1111/j.1600-0404.2008.01014.x] [PMID: 18384454]

[108] Yoneda Y, Okuda S, Hamada R, *et al.* Hospital cost of ischemic stroke and intracerebral hemorrhage in Japanese stroke centers. Health Policy 2005; 73(2): 202-11.
[http://dx.doi.org/10.1016/j.healthpol.2004.11.016] [PMID: 15978963]

[109] Qureshi AI, Suri MF, Nasar A, *et al.* Changes in cost and outcome among US patients with stroke hospitalized in 1990 to 1991 and those hospitalized in 2000 to 2001. Stroke 2007; 38(7): 2180-4.
[http://dx.doi.org/10.1161/STROKEAHA.106.467506] [PMID: 17525400]

[110] Andrew NE, Thrift AG, Cadilhac DA. The prevalence, impact and economic implications of atrial fibrillation in stroke: what progress has been made? Neuroepidemiology 2013; 40(4): 227-39.
[http://dx.doi.org/10.1159/000343667] [PMID: 23364221]

[111] Arboix A, García-Eroles L, Massons JB, Oliveres M, Pujades R, Targa C. Atrial fibrillation and stroke: clinical presentation of cardioembolic *versus* atherothrombotic infarction. Int J Cardiol 2000; 73(1): 33-42.
[http://dx.doi.org/10.1016/S0167-5273(99)00214-4] [PMID: 10748308]

[112] Paciaroni M, Agnelli G, Caso V, *et al.* Atrial fibrillation in patients with first-ever stroke: frequency, antithrombotic treatment before the event and effect on clinical outcome. J Thromb Haemost 2005;

3(6): 1218-23.
[http://dx.doi.org/10.1111/j.1538-7836.2005.01344.x] [PMID: 15892862]

[113] Brüggenjürgen B, Rossnagel K, Roll S, *et al.* The impact of atrial fibrillation on the cost of stroke: the Berlin acute stroke study. Value Health 2007; 10(2): 137-43.
[http://dx.doi.org/10.1111/j.1524-4733.2006.00160.x] [PMID: 17391422]

[114] Ghatnekar O, Glader E-L. The effect of atrial fibrillation on stroke-related inpatient costs in Sweden: a 3-year analysis of registry incidence data from 2001. Value Health 2008; 11(5): 862-8.
[http://dx.doi.org/10.1111/j.1524-4733.2008.00359.x] [PMID: 18489491]

[115] Meretoja A, Kaste M, Roine RO, *et al.* Direct costs of patients with stroke can be continuously monitored on a national level: performance, effectiveness, and Costs of Treatment episodes in Stroke (PERFECT Stroke) Database in Finland. Stroke 2011; 42(7): 2007-12.
[http://dx.doi.org/10.1161/STROKEAHA.110.612119] [PMID: 21527757]

[116] Prepared for the National Stroke Foundation. PricewaterhouseCoopers: The Economic Costs of Atrial Fibrillation in Australia 2010.

[117] Luengo-Fernandez R, Gray AM, Rothwell PM. A population-based study of hospital care costs during five years after TIA and stroke. Author manuscript; available in PMC 15 July 2016. Published in final edited form in. Stroke 2012; 43(12): 3343-51.
[http://dx.doi.org/10.1161/STROKEAHA.112.667204] [PMID: 23160884]

[118] Niemi ML, Laaksonen R, Kotila M, Waltimo O. Quality of life 4 years after stroke. Stroke 1988; 19(9): 1101-7.
[http://dx.doi.org/10.1161/01.STR.19.9.1101] [PMID: 3413807]

[119] Low JT, Kersten P, Ashburn A, George S, McLellan DL. A study to evaluate the met and unmet needs of members belonging to Young Stroke groups affiliated with the Stroke Association. Disabil Rehabil 2003; 25(18): 1052-6.
[http://dx.doi.org/10.1080/0963828031000069753] [PMID: 12944160]

[120] Banks P, Pearson C. Parallel lives: younger stroke survivors and their partners coping with crisis. Sex Relationship Ther 2004; 19: 413-29.
[http://dx.doi.org/10.1080/14681990412331298009]

[121] Röding J, Lindström B, Malm J, Ohman A. Frustrated and invisible--younger stroke patients' experiences of the rehabilitation process. Disabil Rehabil 2003; 25(15): 867-74.
[http://dx.doi.org/10.1080/0963828031000122276] [PMID: 12851097]

[122] Kersten P, Low JT, Ashburn A, George SL, McLellan DL. The unmet needs of young people who have had a stroke: results of a national UK survey. Disabil Rehabil 2002; 24(16): 860-6.
[http://dx.doi.org/10.1080/09638280210142167] [PMID: 12450462]

[123] Teasell RW, McRae MP, Finestone HM. Social issues in the rehabilitation of younger stroke patients. Arch Phys Med Rehabil 2000; 81(2): 205-9.
[http://dx.doi.org/10.1016/S0003-9993(00)90142-4] [PMID: 10668776]

[124] Sjögren K, Fugl-Meyer AR. Adjustment to life after stroke with special reference to sexual intercourse and leisure. J Psychosom Res 1982; 26(4): 409-17.
[http://dx.doi.org/10.1016/0022-3999(82)90015-0] [PMID: 7143281]

[125] Mackay A, Nias BC. Strokes in the young and middle-aged: consequences to the family and to society. J R Coll Physicians Lond 1979; 13(2): 106-12.
[PMID: 439043]

[126] Sjögren K. Leisure after stroke. Int Rehabil Med 1982; 4(2): 80-7.
[http://dx.doi.org/10.3109/09638288209166884] [PMID: 7174217]

[127] Jennum P, Iversen HK, Ibsen R, Kjellberg J. Cost of stroke: a controlled national study evaluating societal effects on patients and their partners. BMC Health Serv Res 2015; 15: 466.
[http://dx.doi.org/10.1186/s12913-015-1100-0] [PMID: 26464109]

[128] Huffman MD, Rao KD, Pichon-Riviere A, *et al.* A cross-sectional study of the microeconomic impact of cardiovascular disease hospitalization in four low- and middle-income countries. PLoS One 2011; 6(6): e20821.
[http://dx.doi.org/10.1371/journal.pone.0020821] [PMID: 21695127]

[129] Okumura Y, Ito H. Out-of-pocket expenditure burdens in patients with cardiovascular conditions and psychological distress: a nationwide cross-sectional study. Gen Hosp Psychiatry 2013; 35(3): 233-8.
[http://dx.doi.org/10.1016/j.genhosppsych.2012.12.013] [PMID: 23391611]

[130] Heeley E, Anderson CS, Huang Y, *et al.* Role of health insurance in averting economic hardship in families after acute stroke in China. Stroke 2009; 40(6): 2149-56.

[131] Banthin JS, Bernard DM. Changes in financial burdens for health care: national estimates for the population younger than 65 years, 1996 to 2003. JAMA 2006; 296(22): 2712-9.
[http://dx.doi.org/10.1001/jama.296.22.2712] [PMID: 17164457]

[132] Essue BM, Hackett ML, Li Q, Glozier N, Lindley R, Jan S. How are household economic circumstances affected after a stroke? The Psychosocial Outcomes In StrokE (POISE) Study. Stroke 2012; 43(11): 3110-3.
[http://dx.doi.org/10.1161/STROKEAHA.112.666453] [PMID: 22949473]

[133] Dewey HM, Thrift AG, Mihalopoulos C, *et al.* Lifetime cost of stroke subtypes in Australia: findings from the North East Melbourne Stroke Incidence Study (NEMESIS). Stroke 2003; 34(10): 2502-7.
[http://dx.doi.org/10.1161/01.STR.0000091395.85357.09] [PMID: 12970517]

CHAPTER 8

Understanding Stroke in a Global Context – Key Points in Plain Language

Shanthi Mendis[*]

Geneva Learning Foundation, Former Senior Adviser World Health Organization, Geneva, Switzerland

The brain is a highly complex organ that requires a regular supply of glucose and oxygen for proper function. Glucose and oxygen are carried to the brain dissolved in blood that runs in blood vessels. Stroke occurs when the blood supply to a part of the brain is interrupted due to obstruction or rupture of a brain blood vessel. Blockage inside blood vessels is caused by accumulation of bad fat and cholesterol in their walls; a process known as atherosclerosis. Less commonly, obstruction to blood supply of the brain may be due to a blood clot that has originated in another part of the body such as the heart. Depending on the cause of interruption to blood supply of the brain, strokes are described as thrombotic, haemorrhagic or embolic.

Atherosclerosis develops due to unhealthy behaviour such as tobacco use, harmful use of alcohol, lack of regular physical activity and consumption of unhealthy diets. Diet is unhealthy when it is too rich in salt, fat and energy (calories) and lacks fruits, vegetables, minerals and fibre. Exposure to polluted air also increases the risk of atherosclerosis.

Unhealthy behaviour results in overweight, obesity, high blood pressure, diabetes and high cholesterol levels in blood. These are additional risk factors that promote atherosclerosis, which leads to stroke.

Stroke is a common illness of the brain that can affect any adult, usually after middle age. Strokes often result in severe disability or death. Strokes are preventable if individual action is supported by public health policies that reduce exposure to risk factors of stroke.

Worldwide, stroke is the second leading cause of death and the third leading cause of disability. Globally, the majority of strokes (70%) and stroke-related deaths

[*] **Corresponding author Shanthi Mendis:** Geneva Learning Foundation, Geneva, Switzerland; Tel/Fax: 0041227880311; E-mail: prof.shanthi.mendis@gmail.com

(87%) occur in low- and middle-income countries. Over the last four decades, the occurrence of stroke (incidence) has more than doubled in low- and middle-income countries, while it has declined in high-income countries.

Strokes, heart attacks, diabetes, cancer and chronic respiratory disease are known as major non-communicable diseases (NCDs). They are caused by the same behavioural and environmental risk factors: tobacco use; harmful use of alcohol; physical inactivity; unhealthy diet; and air pollution. The more risk factors a person has, the greater the risk of strokes and other NCDs. Often people are affected by more than one NCD. For example, stroke and diabetes often occur together because they share the same risk factors.

Power, profit and politics are forces that drive the exposure of people to tobacco use, harmful use of alcohol, physical inactivity and unhealthy diet.

Governments have the responsibility and a fundamental role to play in protecting people from exposure to behavioural and environmental risk factors. Supportive policy environments make healthy choices and behaviours easier, and unhealthy choices and behaviours more difficult.

To prevent stroke (NCDs), people need to be protected from exposure to behavioural and environmental risk factors through strong public health policies. For example, policies to control tobacco and alcohol use, conducive environments for physical activity and affordable fruits and vegetables promote healthy behaviour. Most of these policies require action from ministries outside of the Ministry of Health such as ministries of finance, trade and agriculture.

Individual action is extremely important and people need to adopt healthy behaviour. Undoubtedly behaviour change is difficult and challenging, but there is a greater chance of people maintaining healthy behaviours if they are in conducive regulatory, legislative, economic and physical environments.

Too often actors with vested interests undermine the development and implementation of public health policies that reduce the exposure of people to risk factors of stroke such as tobacco, alcohol, unhealthy diet and physical inactivity. The tobacco, alcohol and food industries consistently use devious tactics to protect profits at the expense of the health of people. Governments and political leaders are responsible for protecting the development and implementation of these policies from parties with vested interests. Civil society should lobby and support governments to develop and implement policies that protect the health of people.

Standards of prevention and care for stroke (NCDs) depend on financial and other resources. Standards of health care for stroke vary tremendously in different countries depending on the level of economic development.

Health systems have a key role in prevention, acute care and rehabilitation of stroke. To prevent the first attacks of stroke, people at high risk of stroke need to be identified in primary care and provided treatment. The detection of people at high risk simply does not happen in countries with weak primary care systems.

In addition, most low-income countries do not have facilities to deliver acute stroke care. Stroke patients must be rapidly identified and transported to appropriate centres that provide optimal treatment as fast as possible.

Nearly two thirds of individuals who develop a stroke either die or are disabled. The chances of dying are much higher with subsequent strokes, which often occur within one year of the first attack. After the first attack of stroke, medicines are required to prevent repeated attacks.

Improving stroke services and treatment can have a major impact on patient outcomes. Hospital-based stroke units can benefit most stroke patients and could be widely implemented. Ideally, all stroke patients would be admitted directly to a stroke unit.

Acute stroke management practice in low-resource settings needs to include supportive care measures such as maintaining the control of blood pressure, blood sugar, body temperature, prevention of clot formation in leg veins and aspiration, and early mobilization and prompt treatment of fits.

Although stroke treatment has advanced significantly over the last two decades and highly effective interventions exist that reduce disability after a stroke, they require much broader implementation to maximize benefit. The majority of stroke victims worldwide currently have no access to high technology stroke interventions because of weak health systems. For patients to benefit from advances in therapy, technology must be embedded in systems that allow rapid treatment because stroke progresses quickly in the first few hours after onset. At present, there is a serious disconnect between advances in the field of stroke and its worldwide application. Most low-income countries do not invest enough in health care to enable implementation of new medical advances for the treatment of stroke such as clot busting therapy.

Stroke (NCDs) cannot be prevented if action is taken only to provide health care for strokes, while exposure to risk factors is ignored. A public health approach to stroke needs to combine policies to reduce exposure to behavioural and environmental risk factors with policies to detect and treat high-risk individuals in primary care. Surveillance and monitoring of these policies are critical for effective implementation.

Despite the fact that stroke risk factors are well known and many prevention strategies are in place, the increasing burden of stroke implies that stroke prevention strategies have not been effectively implemented worldwide. To prevent stroke (NCDs), countries need to strengthen their ability to overcome barriers driven by power, profits and politics that prevent the implementation of health promotion policies.

At a minimum, the utmost priority must be accorded to primary and secondary prevention of stroke in low- and middle-income countries. Basic interventions for prevention and treatment of stroke need to be incorporated in essential service packages of universal health coverage schemes.

Stroke has a large adverse impact on macroeconomic productivity and national and household income and poses a significant financial burden on health-care budgets.

There are considerable differences in costs from productivity loss due to stroke between countries. There is also likely to be a differential impact of stroke on economic productivity in high-income and low- and middle-income countries because case fatality and disability rates are higher in these countries compared to high-income countries.

The estimated global economic loss due to cardiovascular disease (stroke and heart disease) was estimated at US$ 863.5 billion in 2010. It is estimated to increase by 22% and rise to US$ 1.04 billion by 2030. For the period 2011–2025, the cumulative lost output in low- and middle-income countries associated with cardiovascular disease is projected to more than US$ 3.76 trillion.

The total cost of implementing a set of highly cost-effective interventions for prevention and management of stroke across all low- and middle-income countries for the period 2011–2025 is estimated at US$ 170 billion. This amounts to an annual per capita investment of under US$ 1 in low-income countries, US$ 1.50 in lower-middle-income countries and US$ 3 in upper-middle- income countries.

Although 82% of the stroke burden is in low- and middle-income countries, the vast majority of studies (96%) investigating the economic impact of stroke are from high-income countries. More research is urgently needed to assess the true economic burden of stroke in low- and middle-income countries.

Worldwide of all major NCDs, stroke, heart disease and cancer have the highest reported mean annual total direct costs. Total direct health-care expenditure on stroke is estimated at 4–6% of National Health Service expenditure in high-income countries. Hospital costs represent the main driver of stroke expenditure, accounting for 90% of total direct costs.

As health financing systems are reformed for achieving universal health coverage, due consideration should be given to cost-effective interventions to prevent and control stroke.

The current staggering and projected economic burden of stroke poses a barrier to sustainable development. Prevention and control of stroke should, therefore, be prioritized with other major NCDs and addressed within the wider development agenda.

The 2030 Agenda for Sustainable Development is an ambitious initiative of the United Nations, with 17 goals and 169 targets, integrating health, economic development, elimination of extreme poverty, social inclusion, environmental sustainability and good governance.

There is a mutually reinforcing relationship between health and the three dimensions of sustainable development – social, economic and environmental. The health status of people is dependent on holistic development, connected by health systems, behavioural, biochemical and environmental risk factors, ecosystems and the social and structural determinants of health, including enabling legal environments, financing and governance.

The 2030 Agenda for Sustainable Development, with direct and indirect health dimensions in all of the Sustainable Development Goals, offers an unprecedented opportunity to adopt a multi-dimensional and multi-sectoral approach to promote health and prevent and control stroke (NCDs). Prevention and control of NCDs should be an integral component of the national Sustainable Development Goals response.

To implement policies to effectively address stroke (NCDs), governments need to reframe prevention and control of stroke (NCDs), shifting from the health sector model to embrace the multi-sectoral model that underpins the 2030 Agenda for Sustainable Development.

The 17 Sustainable Development Goals focus on: poverty; hunger; health; education; gender equality; water and sanitation; energy; economic growth and employment; industry, innovation and infrastructure; inequality; sustainable cities; consumption and production; climate change; marine resources; terrestrial ecosystems; peace, justice and accountability; and global partnership for sustainable development. Since all these issues are interlinked they cannot be effectively addressed through isolated vertical approaches.

Sustainable Development Goal 3 addresses all major health priorities, including stroke and other NCDs, which is integral for the attainment of all of the goals.

In many low- and middle-income countries, the information infrastructure needs to be strengthened to collect and use all the data required for the indicators of the 2030 Agenda for Sustainable Development.

The Sustainable Development Agenda presents a unifying platform which can advance social and economic development while safeguarding the health and wellbeing of the planet and its people. It is a momentous opportunity to bring all countries and citizens together to take transformative steps to rid people of preventable diseases such as stroke and to shift the future of the world to a sustainable and resilient development path.

CONFLICT OF INTEREST

The author declares no conflict of interest, financial or otherwise.

ACKNOWLEDGEMENTS

Ms AvisAnne Julien is thanked for copy-editing.

SUBJECT INDEX

A

Absolute risk 55, 69

Activities 31, 32, 122, 124, 126
  diet and physical 31
  health promotion 32
  human 122, 124, 126

Acute stroke 12, 14, 15, 16, 34, 35, 68, 94, 102, 110, 113, 139, 148, 149, 152, 165
  care unit 110
  cost 149
  interventions 15
  management practice in low-resource settings 165

Affluent provinces 149

Agenda for sustainable development 36, 98, 99, 100, 124, 130, 167, 168

Air pollution 1, 6, 15, 19, 104, 105, 119, 124, 164
  indoor 6, 124

Albumin 34, 89

Alcohol industries 21, 130

Alcohol use 1, 2, 5, 7 , 10, 13, 15, 19, 25, 30, 31, 32, 36, 41, 42, 52, 54, 164
  harmful 1, 2, 5, 7, 10, 15, 19, 30, 31, 36, 41, 42, 52, 54, 164

Allied health staffing levels 75

Aneurysms 9, 74

Annual stroke-attributable DALY count 143

Anticoagulants 12, 13, 65

Antiplatelet agents 12, 65, 66

Asymptomatic carotid stenosis 56, 57, 58

Atherosclerosis 1, 3, 4, 10, 55, 56, 163
  carotid 55, 56

Atrial fibrillation 4, 6, 13, 15, 66, 139, 149, 150
  -related stroke 149, 150
  -related stroke costs 150

Avoiding heart attacks 3, 4

B

Basel convention 122

Behavioural risk factors 2, 5, 10, 19, 20, 32, 41, 52, 53, 54, 58, 129

Behaviours 20, 21, 24, 25, 34, 108, 163
  health-harming 108
  unhealthy 20, 163
  unhealthy consumption 21, 24, 25, 34

Biodiversity loss 126, 127

Blood 1, 2, 3, 4, 10, 11, 12, 14, 35, 55, 67, 71, 73, 74, 75, 87, 89, 163
  clots 1, 4, 12, 35, 73, 89, 163
  fats 10, 14
  flow 1, 2, 3, 11, 55, 67, 71, 74, 75, 87

Blood pressure 6, 7, 9, 12, 53, 63, 66, 73, 163
  diastolic 9
  high 6, 7, 9, 12, 66, 163
  lowering 8, 63, 73
  systolic 9, 53

Brain blood vessel 1, 163

Brain imaging 63, 67, 69, 68, 70, 71
  advanced 69, 70

Brains, normal 69, 73

Brain tissue 2, 3, 67, 71, 81

C

Capabilities, technological 115, 116

Capacity 27, 30, 105
  health sector 105
  inadequate 27
  national 30

Capacity assessment survey, global 34

Capacity-building 123, 131

Carbon dioxide 122, 124

Cardiovascular disease 2, 36, 53, 104, 119, 139, 140, 141, 142, 148, 166

Cardiovascular disease risk 53, 54
  evaluating absolute 53
  moderate 53

Cardiovascular risk factor control 55

Caring for stroke survivors 52

Carotid endarterectomy 41, 55, 56, 57, 58, 86

Carotid revascularization 57

Carotid stenosis 56, 57, 58